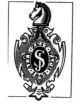

J. Papillon

Rectal and Anal Cancers

Conservative Treatment
by Irradiation –
an Alternative to Radical Surgery

Foreword by O. H. Beahrs

With 35 Figures and 6 Color Plates

Springer-Verlag
Berlin Heidelberg New York 1982

Jean Papillon, M. D.
Professor of Radiology
University of Lyon,
Head of Radiotherapy Department,
Centre Léon Bérard
F-69008 Lyon

ISBN-13:978-3-642-68615-3   e-ISBN-13:978-3-642-68613-9
DOI: 10.1007/978-3-642-68613-9

Library of Congress Cataloging in Publication Data.
Papillon, Jean.
Rectal and anal cancers.
Bibliography: p.
Includes index.
1. Rectum – Cancer – Radiotherapy. 2. Anus – Cancer – Radiotherapy. I. Title. [DNLM:
1. Anus neoplasms – Radiotherapy. 2. Rectal neoplasms – Radiotherapy. WI 610 P 216r]
RC 280. R 37 P 36   1982   616. 99'4350642   82-10805
ISBN-13:978-3-642-68615-3 CU.S.)

This work is subject to copyright. All rights are reserved, whether the whole or part of the material is concerned, specifically those of translation, reprinting, re-use of illustrations, broadcasting, reproduction by photocopying machine or similar means, and storage in data banks. Under § 54 of the German Copyright Law where copies are made for other than private use a fee is payable to "Verwertungsgesellschaft Wort", Munich.

© by Springer-Verlag Berlin Heidelberg 1982
Softcover reprint of the hardcover 1st edition 1982

The use of general descriptive names, trade marks, etc. in this publication, even if the former are not especially identified, is not to be taken as a sign that such names, as understood by the Trade Marks and Merchandise Marks Act, may accordingly by used freely by anyone.

2124/3140-543210

*To Dr. Rupert B. Turnbull jr.,
surgeon at the Cleveland Clinic,
who gave me much help and
encouragement in the
writing of this monograph.*

Foreword

Although attempts at radical removal of cancers of the rectum had been performed earlier, it was not until W. E. Miles in 1908 reported his experience in the management of cancer in this anatomic part, that the combined abdominoperineal resection became the recognized and accepted approach for the treatment of this cancer. Miles reasoned that proctectomy removed the cancer, bearing a segment of large bowel but also the regional lymphatics into which the cancer spread, not only proximally, but laterally and distally as well. In his monograph in 1926 he stated:

...There are, I hold, two main principles to be observed in the surgical treatment of cancer of the rectum and indeed of all cancers wherever they are found, first, operation should be based on a knowledge of the demonstrable facts of pathology, and, second, the most extensive operation possible in conformity with that knowledge should be performed on all patients no matter how small or early the local manifestation of the disease may seem to be...

This philosophy was appropriate in his time but today, with increased knowledge regarding the biological behavior of cancer of the rectum, the recognition of the importance of the extent of the primary lesion and staging of cancer, and the availability of multiple modalities in the management of neoplastic disease, the philosophy has appropriately changed.

Previously, local treatment of cancers of the rectum was associated with a high incidence of failure or recurrence, and the mortality and morbidity associated with resection and an intra-abdominal anastomosis was unacceptably high. So, for the early part of the twentieth century, the combined abdominoperineal resection of the rectum in one or multiple stages remained almost the sole method of treatment of cancer of the rectum. Although radiation treatment was used after its discovery and since the 1920s, it did not prove to be the panacea hoped for, largely because of lack of sophistication in its use and its application most often for advanced lesions.

The overall mortality rate for colon and rectal surgery was 20% or greater until the decades of the thirties and forties. When chemotherapeutic agents and, later, antibiotics became available for preoperative bowel preparation and the treatment of infections, the mortality rate gradually dropped to 5%. Today rates of 2% are frequently reported. With improved safety of colon and rectal surgery, lesser procedures were again tried. Anterior resection has become the procedure of choice for cancers of the lower sigmoid, rectosigmoid, most lesions of the upper one third and some lesions of the mid third of the rectum. This procedure eliminates the need of a permanent colostomy. If normal anatomy and bowel function can be preserved without reducing the chance of cure, the patient is well served. It is unfortunate, though, if a lesser procedure has been carried out to prevent a colostomy resulting in inadequate treatment of a cancer. However, it is also unfortunate if a colostomy is the result of treatment and in creating it, the colostomy has not contributed to the cure of the cancer.

For cancers of the lower one third of the rectum and many of the mid-rectum, the combined abdominoperineal resection is the only feasible radical operation, from the technical standpoint, to remove a cancer. This always means a colostomy. Dukes in 1932 recognized that a cancer goes through stages in its growth, and in his report classified cancers as Stage A when localized to the rectal wall, B when through the wall but without regional lymph node involvement, and C when regional lymph node metastases are present. The Dukes' classification has been modified by many, and other staging recommendations have been made, but the original classification by Dukes remains the simplest and possibly the best. If a surgical specimen is available after radical resection, then accurate pathologic staging can be determined. Unfortunately, on clinical grounds, there is an error in classifying a lesion accurately. In about 10% to 12% of cases of cancer of the rectum clinically considered to be Dukes Stage A or B, regional node metastasis will be present. In all lesions about 50% will have associated nodal metastasis. In arriving at a judgement as to treatment, this error must be kept in mind.

Excision, electrocoagulation, cryosurgery, and intracavitary irradiation have all been shown to destroy primary lesions of the rectum. Therefore, if cancers of the lower rectum are properly selected as most likely being in situ lesions or Dukes A or B, then conservative treatment is reasonable to consider. Results can be excellent. For example, assuming only a 10% error in clinical staging with destruction of the primary lesion, 90% of patients should be cured. If patients so treated are followed carefully, and if the conservative measures should fail or if regional disease becomes apparent, a radical operation can still be done, with frequent favorable results. In patients with more advanced lesions of the rectum in whom there is medical disease increasing significantly the risk of anesthesia and surgical, conservative treatment can be used. If the primary lesion is successfully treated, about 50% should survive the cancer, since approximately that number of patients will have localized disease.

Foreword

The type of conservative treatment is not necessarily all-important in curing selected lesions. Excision should remove the entire gross lesion and this has advantage in that the whole tumor is available for the pathologic study. If fulguration or intracavitary irradiation is to be used, either total excision on a small lesion should be done as a biopsy, or at least an adequate extensive biopsy done, so pathologically the tumor can be staged as accurately as possible. While excision and fulguration frequently require hospitalization on one or several occasions, the use of intracavitary irradiation does not. Because of the high cost of medical care, this becomes an important factor in deciding in favour of one method of treatment versus another, assuming each has equal results.

The author, Jean Papillon, in this treatise nicely discusses the biological behavior of cancer of the rectum and anus, the staging of cancer, and the proper selection of cases for less than radical treatment. As a proponent of intracavitary irradiation treatment of selected cases of cancer of the rectum, he has established his position very well with solid data and sound judgement. Likewise, he extends his thinking to the management of epidermoid carcinoma of the anal and perianal region. Also included is information on the appropriate place of radiation therapy as an additive to surgery or as a part of multiple-modality approach to the treatment of cancer.

Dr. Papillon through his research and clinical experience has contributed greatly to the understanding of the behavior of cancer of the rectum and anus, to the appropriate management of those lesions by less than radical surgical procedures, and in particular by the use of intracavitary irradiation. Most importantly, he has contributed to an improved quality of life for many patients with neoplastic disease of the distal large intestine.

Rochester, June 1982   Oliver H. Beahrs
Professor of Surgery, Emeritus
Mayo Medical School
Consultant, Department of Surgery
(retired)
Mayo Clinic
Rochester, Minnesota, USA

Preface

This monograph is the result of my experience in the management of cancer of the rectum and anus at the Centre Léon Bérard, Lyon, during the past 30 years. In the early years, irradiation made only a small contribution to the conservative treatment of these diseases, and surgeons were reluctant to refer their patients for treatment because there was little experience in this field. Since then there has been a great increase in our knowledge of the natural history of these tumours and their response to irradiation.

Carefully controlled schedules of irradiation (external or intracavitary) have now been developed which are capable of curing certain tumours of the rectum and the anus. The tumours must be selected according to strict criteria, which will be described in this monograph. Only a small proportion of rectal adenocarcinomas are suitable for conservative irradiation, whereas a high proportion of squamous cancers of both anal canal and margin respond to this modality of treatment.

It must be emphasized that the radiotherapist has joint clinical responsibility with the surgeon for the decisions about the conservative treatment of rectal and anal cancers. Both clinicians must consider the individual needs of each patient, and evaluate the respective roles of radiotherapy and surgery to define the best approach in each case in an atmosphere of mutual respect and confidence.

I wish to express my deep gratitude to Mr. Christopher Marks, surgeon in Guildford, Surrey, England, for his patience and devotion in correcting the manuscript of this monograph, and for the constructive advice which he afforded me.

I would also like to thank Dr. Pierre Chapuis, surgeon in Sydney, Australia, whose help was greatly appreciated, and Dr. Danielle Jaussaud, radiotherapist in Lyon, who undertook the considerable task of compiling the bibliography.

Lyon, July 1982   Jean Papillon

Table of Contents

Introduction 1

Section A. Carcinoma of the Rectum 3

I. General Considerations 5
1. Age and Sex Distribution 6
2. Topographical Distribution 6
3. Stage Distribution 6

II. Pathology 8
1. Histology 8
2. Natural History 9
3. Spread of Rectal Cancer 11
   a) Local 11
   b) Lymphatic 13
   c) Venous 16
   d) Distant Metastases 17
4. Staging 17

III. Surgical Treatment 19
1. Criteria Governing Choice of Procedure 19
2. Surgical Results 20
   a) Operative Mortality 22
   b) Sequelae of Surgery 23
3. Additional Therapy 23
   a) Pre-operative Irradiation 24
   b) Pre-operative Chemotherapy and Radiotherapy
      Combined 32
   c) Post-operative Irradiation 33

IV. Rationale of Conservative Treatment for Cure 39
1. Selection of Suitable Cases 40
   a) Risk of Lymphatic Spread 40
   b) Site of Tumour 49
   c) Status of Patient 50
2. Proper Schedules for Treatment 51
3. Follow-up 51
4. Modalities of Conservative Treatment for Rectal Cancer 52

V. Conservative Treatment by Surgery 53
1. Local Excision 53
2. Electrocoagulation 56
   a) Results 57
3. Cryosurgery 61

VI. Conservative Treatment by Irradiation 63
1. Historical Background 63
2. External Beam Irradiation 65
3. Intracavitary Irradiation of Rectal Tumours 66
   a) Contact X-ray Therapy 66
   b) Interstitial Curietherapy 70
   c) Development of Intracavitary Irradiation 75
   d) Experience at the Centre Léon Bérard (Papillon) . . . 77
   e) Problem of Rectal Adenocarcinomas
      of the Juxta-anal Area 95
   f) Indications 98

**VII. Comparison of Surgical and Radiotherapeutic Methods
of Local Therapy** 100
1. Mode of Action 100
2. Conditions of Application 101
3. Control of Tumour 101
4. Follow-up 103
5. Conclusion 103

**VIII. Intracavitary Irradiation as a Supplementary Procedure
After Local Excision – Problem of Villous Adenomas** 104
1. Experience at the Centre Léon Bérard 105

Section B. Epidermoid Carcinoma of the Anus 107

Topographical Distribution of Anal Cancers 109

IX. Epidermoid Carcinoma of the Anal Canal 110
1. Introduction 110
2. Anatomical and Pathological Background 111

X. General Features 114
1. Frequency and Sex Distribution 114
2. Age 114
3. Site 114
4. Configuration 115
5. Tumour Spread 116
   a) Local Spread 116
   b) Regional Spread 117
   c) Distant Spread 121
6. Symptoms and Diagnosis 121

7. Pre-treatment Evaluation 122
8. Clinical Staging 124

XI. Treatment 126
1. Surgery 126
   a) Local Excision 126
   b) Major Surgery 127
   c) Extended Surgery 130
   d) Colostomy 130
2. Radiation Therapy 130
   a) Historical Background 131
   b) Interstitial Curietherapy 132
   c) External Beam Irradiation with Cobalt-60 135
   d) Complications of Irradiation 136

XII. New Therapeutic Approaches 138
1. Background 138
   a) Accessibility 138
   b) Radiosensitivity 138
   c) Radionecrosis 139
   d) Time Factor 139
   e) Multimodality Treatment 140
2. Recent Developments 140
   a) Pre-operative Irradiation With or Without
      Chemotherapy 141
   b) Split-course Irradiation 143

XIII. Experience at the Centre Léon Bérard 145
1. First Protocol – Association of Cobalt-60 and
   Iridium-192 Implant in a Split Course 146
2. Second Protocol – Irradiation Followed by Radical
   Surgery 154
3. Third Protocol – Whole-pelvic and Anal Irradiation ... 156
4. Results 157
   a) Curative Irradiation with Cobalt-60 and Iridium-192 . 158
   b) Pre-operative Irradiation and Radical Surgery 160
   c) Whole-pelvic Irradiation for Unresectable Tumours . 161
5. Lymphatic Spread 162
   a) Inguinal Metastasis 162
   b) Pelvic Node Metastasis 164

XIV. Indications for Treatment 171
1. Management of Tumours of the Anal Canal 171
2. Management of Lymph Node Metastasis 172
   a) Inguinal Lymph Nodes 172
   b) Pelvic Lymph Nodes 175

XV. Epidermoid Carcinoma of the Anal Margin 178
1. General Features 178
2. Local Spread 179
3. Clinical Staging 179
4. Treatment 180
   a) Local Excision 180
   b) Irradiation 181
5. Indications 184
   a) Treatment of Tumours of the Anal Margin 184
   b) Treatment of Inguinal Nodes 185

XVI. Conclusion 186

XVII. References 189
   A. Cancer of the Rectum 189
   B. Cancer of the Anus 195

XVIII. Subject Index 199
   A. Cancer of the Rectum 199
   B. Cancer of the Anus 200

Introduction

At the present time, more and more attention is being paid to the policy of conservative treatment for tumours usually treated by radical measures. This is so in the case of tumours of the larynx, of the breast, of the limbs, and more recently of the rectum and anus. Such trends are designed to give each patient not only a good chance of control of his disease, but also an improved quality of life. However, malignant tumours are known to spread into surrounding tissues and regional lymph nodes, and the principle of cancer surgery consists of a wide excision of the site of the primary tumour together with tissues bearing lymph nodes. Therefore controversy has developed between the staunch defenders of the systematic radical approach and the protagonists of a more selective conservative approach. Conservative treatment may be considered only if the following conditions are met:

1. The cure rate after conservative treatment must be at least equal to that following the radical procedures.
2. The preservation of the organ must be complete from both the anatomical and functional points of view.
3. In cases of failure of conservative attempts, subsequent surgery must be able to be performed without giving rise to a high incidence of complications.

The discovery of carcinoma of the rectum usually means that the patient will be submitted to radical surgery – an anterior resection if the tumour is located in the upper part of the rectum, an abdominoperineal (AP) excision with permanent colostomy for many tumours located in the middle rectum and for all tumours of the lower rectum. The justification for such radical surgery is the chance of cure even in the cases in which there has been dissemination to the regional lymph nodes. The results of these radical operations, which are often performed without giving any consideration to the size of the tumour, have made surgeons critical of more limited procedures, for they have considered cure of the disease to be more important than the burden of a permanent colostomy.

A better knowledge of the natural history of rectal adenocarcinoma and the concept that the theoretical advantage of radical surgery may be offset by the mortality attending the procedure have made it clear that local treatment of some rectal cancers is justified in carefully selected patients. It will be shown that intracavitary irradiation has several advantages compared with local excision or electrocoagulation, and deserves an appreciable place in this particular field.

Mention will be made of the role of radiation therapy as adjuvant procedure in the treatment of rectal cancers suitable for radical surgery.

Squamous cell carcinomas of the anal canal are still treated by the same radical procedure as adenocarcinomas of the lower rectum in many institutions. This policy fails to take into consideration the differences in nature and response to radiation between squamous tumours of the anus and adenocarcinomas of the rectum. There have been many developments in the field of radiation therapy during the last 2 decades. New protocols have been designed which will cure a large proportion of patients with anal canal cancer and spare most of them a permanent colostomy, and these will be described.

The place of irradiation in the management of epidermoid carcinomas of the anal margin will also be discussed in comparison with that of surgery, and it will be demonstrated that carefully planned protocols of radiotherapy are able to control the disease in most cases without giving rise to complications.

The principal aim of this monograph is to distinguish those types of tumour of the rectum and anus which can be cured by irradiation without impairment of continence, and to define the most reliable treatment policies.

Section A
Carcinoma of the Rectum

I. General Considerations

In western countries, growths of the large bowel rank second only to those of the lung as a cause of death from cancer. The highest rates for large-bowel cancer are found in North America and New Zealand, the lowest in African and Asian countries (Japan, India, and Singapore).

In the United States, according to the data from the National Cancer Institute's Surveillance, Epidemiology, and End Results Program (American Cancer Society, 1979), colorectal cancers represented 14% of all cancers in men and 15% in women, excluding non-melanoma skin cancers, and were responsible for 12% of cancer deaths in men and 15% in women. The age-adjusted cancer death rate has remained static in men, but has decreased in women from 20% to 15% during the same period.

In France, 15 443 men and women were registered as having died from cancer of the colon and rectum in 1976. Of these cancer deaths the large-bowel tumours represent 13%, 10.8% in men and 16% in women respectively.

These figures should be borne in mind if one considers that cancers of the rectum excluding the rectosigmoid junction represent approximately one-third of large-bowel cancers. In the United States in 1979, 35 000 cases of rectal cancer were expected, 19 000 in men and 16 000 in women, the male preponderance becoming more pronounced after 65 years of age. In England and Wales in 1971, 5 000 men and women died of rectal cancer. GOLIGHER (1977) reported that cancer of the rectum comprised 38% of all cancers of the large bowel in Great Britain. A similar frequency of 42% was reported by Moss and AXTELL (1970) from a large multicentre study of 42 652 large-bowel cancers.

To summarize, if one studies the world-wide distribution of rectal cancer, the age-standardized incidence per 100 000 in western countries according to WATERHOUSE et al. (1976) is, for instance:

	Male	Female
Connecticut, USA	18.2	11.1
New York State, USA	13.7	8.7
Oxford, England	13.1	8.0
Geneva, Switzerland	13.8	8.0

1. Age and Sex Distribution

Carcinoma of the rectum (defined as tumours arising in the distal 15 cm of the large bowel) is a disease of old people. Only 5% of those suffering from the complaint will be less than 45 years of age, and 1% under 30, while 58% are 65 or older. GOLIGHER (1977) found that more than half of his cases were over the age of 60. Therefore a large group of patients are older than 75 and the majority of patients are elderly and at increased risk under radical surgery. Cancer of the rectums is more frequently found among men than women, but this difference has diminished over the last 30 years, from a male–female case ratio of 1 : 4 in 1940–1949 to 1 : 2 in 1965–1969 (AXTELL et al. 1972).

2. Topographical Distribution

It is customary to divide the rectum into three segments: the upper third, from the rectosigmoid junction 15 cm above the anal verge to 11 cm; the middle third, from 11 cm to 6 cm; and the lower third, which encompasses the distal 6 cm and the anal canal. DUKES (1940) found that 30.8% of the growths were located in the upper third, 32.6% in the middle third, and 36.6% in the lower third. These figures were accurate, since they were derived from the study of 1000 operative specimens. For the clinician the location of a tumour is much less accurate. In practice, the majority of tumours are located in the lower half of the rectum and within easy reach of the examining finger.

3. Stage Distribution

The stage distribution of cancer of the rectum at the time of diagnosis remained rather static from the 1950s up to 1970, with 85% of tumours having invaded the perirectal fatty tissues or the lymph nodes, and only 15% of tumours still confined to the rectal wall, without nodal involvement (MORSON 1977).

In 1972 AXTELL et al. reported that in the United States over 45% of all rectal cancers are diagnosed in a localized stage of disease (no nodes involved). The proportion of patients with regional disease (nodes involved) has fluctuated between 27% and 30% since 1950, while the proportion of patients with distant spread of disease has remained at about 20%. AXTELL et al. (1972) reported that 72% of all rectal cancers were treated by surgery alone. Of this group of surgically treated cancers, 53% were diagnosed as localized (no node involved), 34% as regional (mesenteric node involved). Among these surgically treated patients, the 5-year survival rate is 70% for the localized stage of disease and 34% for the regional stage. The 10-year survival rates are 63% for localized cancers and 25% for regional cancers.

Various clinical, social, and anatomical factors should be considered before deciding on the method of treatment. For example, one may have a robust, middle-aged patient or an elderly patient with physical or mental impairments; a large, extensive tumour or a limited rectal cancer; a highly malignant carcinoma or a slowly growing tumour.

All these factors represent a variety of problems which should be dealt with in different ways, and there is need for a more extensive therapeutic repertoire in treating certain borderline cases, rather than selecting a treatment policy based principally on the site of the primary tumour, as has been done in the past.

It is likely that the progress in the early detection of the rectal cancer, that has been made in most western countries, with systematic check-ups and the use of the Haemoccult test in mass screening programmes, will result in a higher detection of patients with early tumours suitable either for restorative resection or more conservative procedures. Improvements in surgical technique have reduced the number of patients treated by abdominoperineal (AP) resection with construction of a permanent colostomy. In the next decade one can expect an increase in the number of patients cured, with better preservation of sphincter function. In the following chapters, stress will be placed on the role of conservative procedures, and especially on that of intracavitary irradiation, in the management of patients with cancer of the rectum.

II. Pathology

Many reviews are now available, covering all aspects of the pathology of rectal carcinoma: DUKES (1960), BACON (1960), GABRIEL (1963), MORGAN (1965), MORSON and BUSSEY (1967), TODD (1968), PARKS (1972) and GOLIGHER (1977).

WATSON and DUKES (1930) have stressed that the most important pathological features of rectal cancer related to prognosis include the histological grade of the tumour, its macroscopic appearance, and the extent of direct spread of the tumour at the time of diagnosis.

1. Histology

The method of surgical treatment is usually based on gross appearance of the tumour, including its site, size and mobility, whilst the histological grade of the tumour is often considered to be of secondary importance.

Four histological types of rectal carcinoma are usually described: (a) well-differentiated or grade I adenocarcinoma; (b) moderately differentiated or grade II adenocarcinoma; (c) poorly differentiated or grade III adenocarcinoma; and (c) colloid carcinoma, which is divided into two subgroups: mucinous carcinoma, with the presence of free mucus; and signet-ring cell carcinoma, where the mucus is stored in individual cells.

It has been said that there are no sharply defined boundaries to the grades of malignancy, and that grading is an artificial division into arbitrary groups. If there is difficulty in categorizing tumours which appear to be of intermediate character, it is easier to divide rectal cancer into two types with different prognoses:

1. Well- and moderately well differentiated carcinomas, or grades I and II (also called low and average grade of malignancy). They represent 80% of cases. They grow slowly and metastasize late. In the series of 2097 cases studied at St. Mark's Hospital, London, the corrected 5-year survival rate was 64.5%.
2. Poorly differentiated adenocarcinomas (grade III) and colloid carcinomas known for their high malignancy. They represent 20% of cases, grow more quickly, and have a great metastasizing potential and a very poor prognosis. The corrected 5-year survival rate was only 28.9%. In 63 cases of colloid carcinoma BACON (1964) reports 69.8% of regional or distant metastases.

There is a relationship between histological grade and local spread. In a series of 985 cases of DUKES (1940), 87% of A cases (confined to the bowel wall, without lymphatic involvement) were histological grade I or II, and only 13% were grade III or colloid. It means that most cancers detected at an early stage, limited to the rectal wall, are of moderate malignancy, which is an additional factor contributing to a better prognosis. The histological type of tumour is also correlated with age, 50% of cancers in patients under 40 being of a high grade of malignancy, whereas in patients over 80, only 11% are of a high grade of malignancy (SANFELIPPO and BEAHRS (1974, SIMSTEIN et al. 1978).

To summarize, from the histological point of view, there are a number of well-recognized features which help to predict the behaviour of rectal cancers. Malignancy is an intrinsic feature of the tumour, and not necessarily related to its size. A small, poorly differentiated tumour, 2 cm in diameter, is much more malignant than a 5-cm well-differentiated adenocarcinoma. This concept must be borne in mind when a decision is made about the appropriate treatment of a tumour. In all cases the histological grade must be accurately assessed. In addition, since the patterns seen on microscopy may vary throughout the tumour, it is preferable to submit multiple biopsies to the pathologist, especially when surgical excision of the tumour is not contemplated.

2. Natural History

At the time of diagnosis, most rectal cancers are ulcerated and infiltrating tumours with evidence of spread through the rectal wall. Much attention has been directed to the natural history of advanced rectal cancer with direct extension to the adjacent pelvic structures and with lymphatic, venous, and metastatic spread. The initial stages of cancer of the rectum deserve more attention from the pathological and clinical points of view.

It is well known that malignant changes may occur in adenomatous polyps and villous adenomas. Several degrees of degeneration have been described: adenomas with atypism, in situ carcinomas, and intramural carcinomas. Although pathologists regard such cases as malignant, GRINNELL and LANE (1958) emphasized that for the clinician only the cases which show invasion through the muscular mucosae can be regarded as true cancer. Carcinoma in a polyp may be found in a small area at the tip of the polyp but may also involve the stalk. In no case will a simple biopsy be adequate, and only the removal of the entire polyp will give the pathologist the opportunity to assess whether malignant change is confined to the polyp.

MORSON (1966) uses the term "early rectal cancer" to describe areas of malignant appearance which have not spread in direct continuity beyond the submucous layer. Between 1948 and 1962, out of a total 2305 rectal cancers treated at St. Mark's Hospital, only 76 (3.3%) came into this category.

A careful histological examination of early cancers may show evidence of a precancerous lesion (MORSON and BUSSEY 1967): benign adenomatous or villous polyps were found in continuity with invasive cancer in 50% of cases. The malignant potential of these benign polyps was related to their size, their histological type, and their degree of epithelial dysplasia. MORSON and BUSSEY (1961) conclude that the polyp–cancer sequence is responsible for the pathogenesis of most, if not all, cancers of the colon and rectum. However, he found associated benign lesions in only 18% of the cancers confined to the rectal wall, and in 10.6% of operative specimens of all rectal cancers in patients treated at St. Mark's Hospital. He emphasizes that the histological expression of increased risk is epithelial dysplasia or atypia, which may arise in a flat mucosa as often as in a polypoid tumour.

This theory of the necessary polyp–cancer sequence is not admitted by HELWIG (1947) and by SPRATT and ACKERMAN (1962), who favour the concept that cancer of the rectum can originate directly from the mucosal surface, without a preliminary polyp. For some authors, it seems difficult to accept that small ulcerative adenocarcinomas less than 15 mm in diameter, or small exophytic cancers without any evidence of a previously innocent lesion, have a benign precursor and are not cancers de novo.

These positions are not so far from each others, since MORSON (1979) admits that "the majority of colorectal cancers have passed through what is now known as the adenoma–carcinoma sequence, but which might more accurately be called the dysplasia–carcinoma sequence". However, the polyp-cancer sequence should be born in mind, because of its implication in the prevention of rectal cancer.

The typical invasive cancer in its early stage is a sessile exophytic mass, dark red or purple, raised above the surrounding mucosa, which is pink, supple, and entirely normal. These malignant polyps, about 2 cm in diameter, have a protruding surface finely or coarsely nodular on most of its extent. They bleed easily on contact after digital examination or rectoscopy. The mass is rather hard by contrast with the surrounding mucosa, and the consistency is not the same in all parts of the tumour. Some areas are softer than others, but induration is always found, especially at the edge of the growth. The lesion feels mobile on the rectal wall to the examining finger (MASON 1977).

There is also a definite border between the tumour and neighbouring mucosa. These malignant polyps may be located at any site in the rectal ampulla. Some are located on the valves, others astride the valves. In any case, their colour and consistency make confusion with benign polyps unlikely.

When a malignant polyp grows, it produces a large fungating mass which projects into the lumen of the bowel, with minimal infiltration of the bowel wall.

After a certain time, malignant polyps become ulcerated. LOCKHART-MUMMERY and DUKES (1952) stated that ulceration usually begins when the muscular layer is reached, due to interference with the blood-supply at the surface and local sepsis. Ulceration is located in the centre of the polyp, which assumes the shape of a crater. At the site of ulceration the tumour is more indurated than at the edge of the lesion; its centre is not necrotic, but dark red. The lesion remains mobile, but not so mobile on the rectal wall as in early tumours.

Later, the ulceration is deeper with sloughing and the crater very indurated. The edges are very hard, and the lesion has an impaired mobility. This demonstrates that the cancer has penetrated through the muscular layer.

Not all rectal tumours have this appearance. Some tumours, in their early stages, appear as flattened, slightly raised buttons in the mucosa without ulceration, or as indurated disc-like lesions elevated as a plateau with a flat though irregular surface and a definite edge. In such cases, the lesion is more infiltrating than protruding into the rectal lumen. The part of the tumour visible at rectoscopy is less important than the hidden part of the lesion. This type of rectal cancer, always hard, is more common in the supra-anal area, where the proximity of the sphincter influences the development of the tumour.

Some rectal cancers, less than 2 cm in diameter, are already ulcerated. They consist of a small circular crater, with raised everted edges, protruding only a few millimeters into the bowel lumen. The ulceration is not very deep and the centre remains dark red, with induration. However, the lesion remains mobile. If it is located on the anterior wall in a female patient, the thickness of a tumour not exceeding ½ cm may easily be appreciated by a combined rectal and vaginal examination.

Sometimes, rectal cancer has the appearance of a sessile lesion similar to a villous tumour. The lesion feels soft, and may be removed as a benign polyp, but be found to be malignant on subsequent histology. Careful clinical examination would have shown a suggestion of induration around its base, which is a reliable sign of malignancy.

There is never any narrowing of the bowel lumen. Any reduction in size of the diameter of the rectal lumen is a sign of the tumour probably having spread through the muscular layer.

3. Spread of Rectal Cancer

Carcinoma of the rectum spreads in three ways: (a) by local extension from its origin, (b) by means of lymphatics, and (c) by venous invasion.

a) Local

Direct spread in continuity is devided into two stages, intramural spread and extramural spread. These stages differ markedly in their prognosis with regard to their potential for regional and distant spread. Two types of rectal cancer are recognized, tumours which are still confined to the rectal wall and tumours which have spread beyond the rectal wall.

Intramural Spread. Starting from a primary focus in the mucosa, the tumour grows in all directions, though usually faster in the transverse than in the longitudinal axis of the bowel. Direct spread in continuity of rectal cancer is usually a slow process, except in highly malignant tumours which do not represent more than 20% of cases. MILES (1926) estimated that invasion of one quadrant of the circumference takes at least 6 months. Accoring to LOYGUE and DUBOIS (1966)

1 year is the estimated time for a tumour to reach 3 cm in diameter, and the same time is necessary for the involvement of the whole depth of the bowel wall. At the time of diagnosis most rectal carcinomas have been developing for a long time.

In the rectal ampulla, polypoid cancers tend to grow large where there is room for them to expand into the lumen. This concept explains why such growths may become rather big (4 cm in diameter) and protrude into the bowel lumen without infiltrating deeply. This rule is not valid for early ulcerative adenocarcinomas, for disc-like tumours, or for cancers arising from the lowest part of the rectum near to the anal canal. The rectal lumen is narrowed and tapered due to the proximity of the sphincter. In this situation rectal tumours protrude less and infiltrate at an earlier stage than lesions located higher in the middle third of the rectum.

On the mucosal aspect the spread of carcinoma appears to end abruptly and is marked by the raised edge of the lesion. Below the mucosa, the tumour invades successively the submucosa and the circular and longitudinal muscular layers.

BLACK and WAUGH (1948) have shown that the spread in the submucosa is characterized by large masses of carcinoma cells pushing the muscular layer away from the mucosa and increasing the thickness of the rectal wall in the region of the tumour. The spread in the muscular layer takes place by incomplete columns of carcinoma cells penetrating down between the muscle bundles.

BACON (1964) has emphasized that the raised edges of the lesion on the mucosa mark the limit of the intramural lesion for grade I and II adenocarcinomas. In his view the surface of the involved mucosa gives a clear idea of the extent of the infiltration of the rectal wall, as long as the primary tumour has not spread beyond the muscular layer and penetrated the perirectal fat.

This idea is not valid for colloid or poorly differentiated carcinomas, which may extend sideways at an early stage beyond the limits of the involved mucosa, nor is it valid for advanced tumours with extension beyond the rectal wall. In such cases, microscopic spread in the rectal wall may be found at a distance of at least 25 mm from the gross tumour.

BACON (1964) does not disagree with the concept that intramural spread is wedge-shaped with the apex at the mucosa and the base in the perirectal fat (MILES 1926). In his comments he is concerned exclusively with tumours confined to the rectal wall.

BACON's ideas are confirmed by our experience with intracavitary contact X-ray therapy. In intracavitary irradiation, a small free margin a few millimeters around the gross lesion is irradiated, and yet the rate of recurrence at the border of the tumour is extremely low.

Extramural Spread. When a rectal cancer spreads beyond the bowel wall, its further progress cannot be predicted. Cancer cells are free to permeate the pararectal fatty tissues, and to invade adjacent structures.

GOLIGHER (1977) has noted that the penetration through the muscle coat begins and is most advanced at a point corresponding to the centre or oldest part of the tumour. Pre-operative irradiation has confirmed this by showing that there is a greater reduction of tumour mass after radiotherapy at the periphery of the lesion and that the residual tumour is located in the centre of the original tumour.

Operative specimens show that more than 80% of rectal cancers have spread beyond the rectal wall at the time of surgical treatment. They are large ulcerative carcinomas, very indurated, with a necrotic centre and a degree of fixity. There is often a certain amount of of stenosis, if not an annular carcinoma. The growth has penetrated through the muscle coat and the neighbouring structures. If the lesion is located in the lower two-thirds, perirectal fat and pelvic structures are invaded. With a growth above the peritoneal reflection, there may be invasion of the serosa, and of adjacent organs such as the small gut, the sigmoid colon, and the urogenital tract, with dissemination of tumour throughout the peritoneal cavity.

Extension through the rectal wall has been graded and DUKES (1960) has described slight, moderate, and extensive extrarectal spread. When a grade I or II rectal cancer penetrates the perirectal tissues, there is only a small increase in size of the tumour. In fact an important event has occurred, and the potential for regional and distant spread has increased significantly.

There is a close relationship between the degree of infiltration of the rectal wall and the cure rate. In the series of DUKES (1960), the crude 5-year survival rate is 81.2% for cases of tumours with intramural spread and 44% for cases of tumours with extramural spread.

Many other studies have confirmed the results at St. Mark's Hospital. One can conclude that there is a lot of difference from the prognostic point of view between rectal cancers still confined to the rectal wall and tumours with extramural spread. The majority of the former may be considered local disease, and the latter extensive disease.

b) Lymphatic

The anatomy of the lymphatics of the rectum has been well described by POIRIER et al. (1903), VILLEMIN et al. (1925), and ROUVIERE (1932). The lymphatic system consists of three main lymphatic trunks, the superior, middle, and inferior, which correspond to the superior, middle, and inferior haemorrhoidal vessels. The superior and main trunks arise from the entire length of the rectum from as low as the anal canal, and drain into the perirectal nodes and afterwards into the nodes situated along the superior haemorrhoidal vessels. The middle trunks arise from the rectum, just above the insertion of the levator ani muscles, and drain into the hypogastric and presacral nodes. The inferior trunks arise from the lowest portion of the rectum and the anal area, and drain chiefly to the inguinal nodes, but also on occasion directly to the iliac and pelvic nodes.

In an important study DUKES and BUSSEY (1950) confirmed that the spread of carcinoma of the rectum through the lymphatics is upward in 99% of cases. They demonstrated that *"the first glands to receive metastases are those situated in the perirectal tissues on the same level, or immediately above the primary growth. The next to be affected are the chain of glands accompanying the superior hemorrhoidal vessels. As a rule these are invaded in sequence from below upwards"*. In all but one of the specimens dissected by the authors, the lymphatic spread has been by such an uninterrupted upwards extension. They stated that *discontinuous spread is*

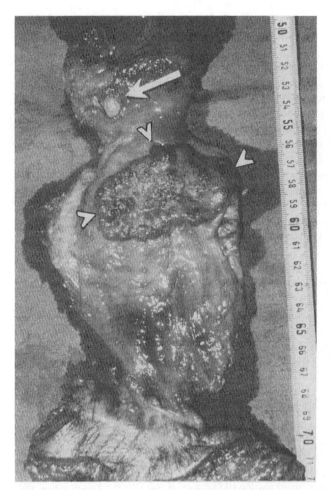

Fig. 1. Operative specimen of AP resection of a patient referred to the radiotherapist for intracavitary irradiation of a polypoid well-differentiated adenocarcinoma of the middle third of the rectum. Before starting irradiation, rectal digital examination showed the presence of a hard nodule in the rectal wall above the primary tumour. The patient was not irradiated and underwent an AP resection. The metastatic lymph node is visible after incision of the rectal mucosa *(white arrow)*. No other metastatic nodes in the specimen

very uncommon. TURNBULL (1974) confirmed that in more than 900 cases the proximal nodes were never involved without satellite node involvement first, and that before a cancer spreads to nodes any distance from the cancer, it must involve the nodes within a centimetre or two around the cancer.

Involved lymph nodes are situated in the mesorectum, in the immediate vicinity of the tumour, attached to the terminal branches of the artery. *For low-lying rectal carcinomas, the first metastatic nodes will therefore be located less than 8 cm from the anal verge, within reach of the examining finger.* Metastatic nodes present as hard mobile nodules, palpable through the rectal wall (Fig. 1).

Involvement of hypogastric nodes is uncommon, but these nodes may be in-

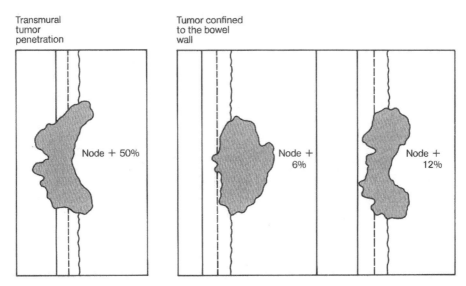

Fig. 2. The probability of lymphatic spread is related to the local spread of a rectal cancer. Tumours which have spread beyond the rectal wall have a high rate of lymph node involvement (50%), whereas well-differentiated adenocarcinomas confined to the rectal wall have a much lower lymphatic risk: 6% in cases of polypoid tomour, 12% in cases of ulcerative tumour

volved by tumours situated in the lower half of the rectum. These metastatic nodes, which are not normally removed in abdominal perineal resection, develop as hard enlarged masses fixed to the pelvic wall. Inguinal lymph nodes may be involved when an adenocarcinoma arises in the anal canal or extends to this area.

The incidence of lymphatic metastases is related to: (a) *degree of histological differentiation,* and (b) local spread. DUKES and BUSSEY (1950) noted, in a series of 2238 operative specimens, that lymphatic involvement occurred more frequently with high-grade or colloid carcinoma (81.3%) than with tumours of low or average malignancy (43.1%). This finding was confirmed by SEEFELD and BARGEN (1943), who showed that the rate of lymphatic spread was 63.6% among patients under 40, who had more poorly differentiated tumours, whereas the rate was lower (28.6%) among the patients over 60 who had better-differentiated adenocarcinomas.

MORSON (1966), in a series of 2084 tumours treated by resection, stressed that there is a close relationship between the rate of lymphatic involvement and the extent of local spread. "For growths spreading in continuity through and beyond the bowel wall, the incidence rises to 58.3%".

By contrast:
with growths limited to the mucosa and submucosa, the rate of lymphatic metastases was 10.9%, exactly 5 in 55 cases, and among these 5 cases, 3 were of a high grade malignancy, and 2 were of an average grade corresponding to BRODERS

Grade III rather than Grade II ... For growths spreading in continuity beyond the submucosa but still confined to the bowel wall, the incidence was 12.1%.

CHOLDINE (1955) found an incidence of 6% of lymphatic metastases when the tumour was limited to the submucosa. MORSON and BUSSEY (1961) concluded that *until penetration of the bowel wall has taken place, the chance of lymphatic metastases having already occurred is very low, as long as the tumour is well – or fairly well differentiated.* This probability may be estimated at 6% for growths limited to the submucosa, and 12% for growths confined to the bowel wall but with spread into the muscular layers (Fig. 2).

Lymphatic spread has a bad prognostic significance. In the series of DUKES (1960) and DUKES and BUSSEY (1950), the crude 5-year survival rate was 65.7% in 1 000 cases without metastatic nodes, and only 27.4% in 1 037 cases with metastatic nodes. In the series of WHITTAKER and GOLIGHER (1976) it was respectively 67% and 33%. The chance of cure in cases with involved nodes was half that of those without metastatic spread.

The number of nodes involved also has an influence on the prognosis. The corrected 5-year survival rate was 63.6% in 125 cases with only one node involved, whereas it was 30% in 439 cases with more than one node involved.

c) Venous

Invasion of the venous channels may produce malignant thrombi with release of malignant emboli which give rise to distant metastases. DUKES (1960) and DUKES and BUSSEY (1950) have shown that the rate of venous invasion was 11% of 1 800 specimens of rectal cancer, although this did not prove that spread to the liver or to the lungs had already occurred.

The most likely place to find evidence of intravascular extension is where the veins emerge from the region of the growth.

A vein containing carcinoma feels hard and nodular. Some times venous nodes of permeation or in-transit metastasis are located very close to the primary growth or a few centimetres above it, and may be discovered by digital examination. Clinically, their induration, their pattern, and their location in the perirectal tissue near to the muscle wall or within the perirectal fat may be the same as those of the metastatic lymph nodes in the mesorectum. Histological examination shows that they do not contain any lymphatic structure, and that they are devoloped in a venous pedicle. Special stains identify them as real veins and not lymphatics.

The incidence of venous invasion increases according to the grade of malignancy and the extent of tumour penetration. In the series of DUKES and BUSSEY (1950), it was only 4.9% with low-grade malignancy but 22.9% for tumours designated as colloid or high-grade tumours. SEEFELD and BARGEN (1943) found 11.7% for grade I and II tumours, and 62.5% for grade III tumours.

No instance of venous spread was found in the A cases (growth limited to the rectal wall). Intravascular invasion was found in 35 of 213 B cases (16.4%). Among the 360 cases in which the lymph glands contained metastases (C cases), DUKES (1960) found 76 (21.1%) with evidence of venous spread. He concluded that the invasion of veins must take place from the primary growth and not as the result of spread from lymphatic metastases because there was so little difference in the incidence of venous spread between B and C cases.

Venous spread is not correlated with such a poor prognosis as lymphatic spread. For DUKES (1960), the corrected 5-year survival rate for those with venous spread was 64%, compared with 32% for those with lymphatic spread. SWINTON et al. (1959) produced similar figures of 60.2% and 36% for both colonic and rectal carcinoma.

d) Distant Metastases

Cancers of the rectum give rise to metastases in the liver or in the lungs – less commonly in bone. These may occur in two circumstances:
1. In highly malignant carcinomas, i.e. poorly differentiated or colloid tumours. In this case metastases are frequent and may develop early (a few months after treatment of the primary lesion or at the time of its discovery), even if the rectal tumour is small.
2. By contrast, metastases from well- or moderately differentiated carcinomas develop late, and most are associated with bulky tumours, with evidence of lymph node spread or with local recurrence after radical surgery.

4. Staging

In oncology, the aim of tumour staging is to allow authors from different institutions and countries to be able to compare their treatment results. Usually, staging is based on clinical data when the tumour is accessible to palpation. Only the lower half of the rectum tumour is accessible to palpation. Only the lower half of the rectum is within reach of the examining finger, and this is the reason why the TNM classification of the UICC, based, for instance, on the degree of infiltration of the muscular coat of the rectum, ist not applicable by the clinician. One of the merits of DUKES has been to propose a pathological staging system based on the examination of operative specimens, which is simple and which has been unanimously accepted. This staging high-lights two principal prognostic factors: local and lymphatic spread. DUKES classification (1932) is as follows:

A cases: Growth limited to rectum; no extrarectal spread; no lymphatic metastases
B cases: Spread by direct continuity into extrarectal tissues; no lymphatic metastases
C cases: Lymphatic metastases present (whatever the degree of local spread).

C cases were further subdivided into two groups to illustrate the extent of lymphatic spread:

C1: Only local nodes contained metastases
C_2 More extensive lymphatic spread involving the nodes at the point of ligature of the blood-vessels.

Several modifications of DUKES classification have been suggested, for instance by ASTLER and COLLER (1954):
A Lesion limited to the mucosa
B_1 Lesion extending into but not through the muscular coat, without positive nodes
B_2 Lesion extending through the muscular coat, without positive nodes
C_1 Lesion limited to the wall, with positive nodes
C_2 Lesion extending through all layers, with positive nodes.

The ASTLER–COLLER (1954) classification is based on the extent of local spread of rectal cancer. In particular, it separates in the group of intramural tumours the superficial from the most infiltrating tumours still confined to the bowel wall. Among the tumours with nodal involvement, this staging separates the intramural and the extramural lesions. In this respect, this classification is more accurate than the DUKES (1932, WATSON and DUKES 1930) classification. Depth of penetration of the rectal wall was a significant prognostic variable independent of lymph node metastases.

The Gastro-Intestinal Tumour Study Group (GITSG) of the National Cancer Institute has defined a third form of staging, which is a modified DUKES classification with six stages:
A Limited to mucosa
B_1 Invasion of muscularis mucosae, submucosa, and muscularis propria
B_2 Invasion of serosa
C_1 One to four lymph nodes involved by tumour
C_2 Five or more lymph nodes involved by tumour
D Distant metastases.

Whatever the type of classification adopted, the stress is always placed on the extent of local spread, and on the significance of nodal involvement.

The numerous staging systems proposed have made it very difficult to compare one report or one series with another. GOLIGHER (1976) has shown that the problem is magnified by the fact that, for some authors, what is termed DUKES classification is quite different from that originally defined. He stressed the need to accept DUKES categorization exactly as it was defined by the author, because it clearly points out the two main criteria related to recurrence and survival: local spread and lymphatic spread.

III. Surgical Treatment

Role of Additional Therapy

1. Criteria Governing Choice of Procedure

In most cases, treatment of cancer of the rectum requires major surgery to remove the primary growth with a large margin of normal bowel beyond the growth and the tissues bearing regional lymph nodes. There is controversy about the relative indications for excisional, sphincter-preserving, and conservative procedures. Radiation therapy may be added to these options as an adjunctive treatment or for cure.

At present, of 100 patients with cancer of the rectum approximately 40 will be alive and well in 5 years' time, but fewer than half of these will have normal anal function and most of the rest will have a permanent colostomy. At least 60 will die from cancer or intercurrent disease within this period. Late diagnosis will permit a maximum of 70–75 patients to be treated radically. The remainder will have palliative treatment because of advanced tumours or poor general health.

When a decision is made about treatment, many different factors must be taken into consideration. MASON (1976a) has said that no two patients with rectal cancer are ever exactly alike, and that there can be no standard operation for every patient with carcinoma of the rectum. Three criteria can be used to classify patients:
  (a) status of the patient,
  (b) extent of the cancer, and
  (c) site of the tumour.

(a) Elderly patients may be obese, senile, and frail, with cardiovascular or respiratory disease, and constitute a very high surgical risk. Young patients aged under 40 with rectal cancer have a higher proportion of poorly differentiated or colloid tumours of poor prognosis than older patients.

(b) As to extent of the cancer, tumours can be separated into four groups:
1. A small group (15%) of limited, highly curable neoplasms
2. A median group of moderately advanced tumours, curable as long as radical surgery is performed with or without pre-operative irradiation (55%–60% of cases)
3. A group of very extensive tumours with or without distant metastasis, only suitable for palliative treatment (about 25% of cases)
4. A group of non-resectable tumours (5%).

(c) The site of tumour is particularly significant for the determination of treatment. The MILES AP resection with permanent colostomy has come to be accepted as the standard orthodox therapy for tumours in the lower half of the rectum. If the tumour is not readily palpable, there are very few circumstances when AP resection is indicated. Anterior resection for lesions above the 10-cm level has been established as the procedure of choice.

In the mid-rectum the choice between these two procedures is often made during surgery, and depends on anatomical relationships and surgical and pathological findings. Factors which modify the decision include the sex of the patient, obesity, pelvic size, and histological grade and size of the tumour.

Recent advances in surgical technique allow a higher proportion of patients with rectal cancer to be spared the inconvenience of a colostomy. Low anterior resection is now applicable to certain tumours of the middle third, even when the inferior border of the lesion is as low as 8 cm from the anal verge.

Various procedures have been developed to allow an anastomosis to be carried out at a low level. Abdominal approach for exposure and mobilization of the rectum may be combined with various transanal, perineal, or sacral techniques to enable a low colorectal or colo-anal anastomosis to be carried out: pull-through procedures (BABCOCK 1947, TURNBULL and CUTHBERTSON 1961, CUGNENC et al. (1981) abdominotransanal resection (PARKS 1972), abdominotranssacral resection (LOCALIO et al. 1978) and transsphincteric operation (MASON 1974, 1980). A special mention must be made of the introduction of new circular stapling devices such as the American EEA instruments, which allow surgeons to perform sphincter-preserving operations for many more patients. These procedures make an end-to-end anastomosis less difficult and allow transection of the rectum far enough beyond the palpable lower edge of the tumour.

PARKS and THOMPSON (1977) have emphasized the necessity of applying such restorative procedures in selected cases for low- or average-grade tumours and tumours which have not extended into the perirectal fat. HERMANEK et al. (1980) has suggested that the surgeon should request frozen sections in these cases in order to:
1. Examine samples of suspect tissue from the peritoneum in order to rule out or verify distant metastases
2. Clarify the relationship of the tumour to neighbouring organs, especially to differentiate between invasive and inflammatory adhesions
3. Check whether the lines of resection are free from tumour.

We do not know whether these restorative methods lead to a difference in the cure rate, but they improve the quality of life by sparing patients the burden of a colostomy.

2. Surgical Results

The results of major surgery in the treatment of carcinoma of the rectum have been analysed in the publications of a number of great surgical centres in western countries. Special mention must be made of the statistics of 3 163 cases operated on at St. Mark's Hospital, reported by LOCKHARDT-MUMMERY et al. (1976), and of the series of 550 cases treated at the General Infirmary, Leeds, reported by WHITTAKER and GOLIGHER (1976).

All the reports emphasize the substantial progress made in the surgery of rectal cancer during the last 3 decades. In the majority of publications, most data are rather similar – but some figures differ markedly. It is generally admitted that the resectability rate is high – about 90% (95% at St. Mark's Hospital). The proportion of operations carried out with a reasonable prospect of cure varies from 60% to 75%, according to the clinical material referred to the hospital. Highly specialized surgical departments have a higher rate of "curable" cases than general hospitals, where emergency large-bowel surgery is more frequent.

The respective proportions of radical operations and restorative operations also differ between centres, ranging from 20% to more than 40%. The 5-year survival rate calculated on immediate operative survivors is about 50% in most institutions, varying from 38.8% to 60%. It is important to distinguish between the "crude" and "corrected" 5-year survival rates. The crude rate is calculated by determining the number of patients still alive after 5 years and expressing it as a percentage of the original series. Crude 5-year survival rate makes no distinction between patients who died of their cancer and patients who died from intercurrent diesase. The corrected 5-year survival rate takes into account the normal expectation of life of the general population of both sexes in different age-groups by means of life-tables. This calculation gives a more accurate picture of the curative value of surgical treatment. The effect of this correction on the figures is to increase the crude survival rate by about one-fifth of its original value for rectal cancer, because most of the patients are elderly.

There is a big difference in the proportion of cases treated by radical and by restorative procedures in several series. This shows that some surgeons rely essentially on AP excision and restrict anterior resection to early tumours of the upper third of the rectum, whereas other surgeons using new procedures for low anastomoses have increased the number of sphincter-saving procedures.

Almost all publications have shown that the chances of cure are better after restorative procedures than after combined AP excision. GOLIGHER (1977) explains this difference by the better prognosis of tumours located in the upper half of the rectum, and by the selection of the lesions and of the patients suitable for sphincter-saving procedures. Highly malignant and extensive tumours of the middle third of the rectum and obese patients are rejected for restorative surgery and relegated to combined excision.

NICHOLLS et al. (1979) studied the long-term results of a total of 199 patients with cancer of the rectum situated between 8 cm and 12 cm from the anal verge, and followed up over 5 years: 112 had been treated by total excision of the rectum, and 87 by restorative operation. There was no significant difference in 5-year survival after either operation when the three pathological variables (grading, DUKES B and DUKES C) are taken into account. They concluded that restorative resection for carcinoma of the mid-rectum is as curative as total excision in terms of 5-year survival.

a) Operative Mortality

The substantial differences in the rates of operative mortality, i.e. the deaths due to complications which occur during the 1st month after surgery, are difficult to explain. In most series, the 5-year survival rates are calculated on the operative survivors, and the end results may be difficult to compare if the operative mortality rates are significantly different.

If one considers the operative death rates reported by several institutions, the figures differ markedly, from 1.7%–2% for centres such as St. Mark's Hospital, the Cleveland Clinic, the Memorial Hospital, and the Mayo Clinic, to a much higher mortality rate in other centres: 10.6% at the General Infirmary in Leeds, 9% in the randomized trial of the European Organization for Cancer Research (1979), 7.6% for RUBAY and BOEUR (1978). In most European centres the operative mortality rate is estimated at between 6% and 8%.

For WHITTAKER and GOLIGHER (1976) these significant differences reflect that some highly specialised hospitals are dealing with a somewhat selectively referred clientèle of patients, who do not represent the outcome of surgical treatment of rectal cancer in other surgical departments, even treated by a staff of surgeons who have a keen interest in colo-rectal surgery. Greater mortality rate reflects the higher proportion of more generally ill patients in some series than those, who are referred to a more specialised hospital.

In all institutions the mortality rate is related to several general condition of the patients, type of operation, and stage of the disease. In many statistical studies no details are given concerning this problem. WHITTAKER and GOLIGHER (1976) give interesting data in this respect. In their series the mortality, usually low, becomes gradually higher in elderly and frail patients. In patients less than 70 years of age it is 7.8%, but rises to 20.5% after 70. The mortality rate is 12.5% after AP resection compared with 7.5% after sphincter-saving procedures. In many series the lethal mishaps are more common after operations for low-lying

Table 1. Results of surgical treatment for rectal cancer (recent series)

Criteria	Average rate	Lowest and highest rates
Resectability	90%	(80% –95%)
Operative mortality	6%	(1.7%– 9%)
Crude 5-year survival	50%	(38.8%–60%)
Curative operations	70%	(65% –80%)
Palliative operations	30%	(20% –40%)
Radical excision	65%	(60% –75%)
Sphincter-saving procedures	35%	(20% –41%)
Crude 5-year survival after radical operation	40%	(34.8%–50%)
Crude 5-year survival after restorative procedures	60%	(45% –65%)
Crude 5-year survival according to the extent of the tumour:		
DUKES A type (15% of cases)	80%	(75% –85%)
DUKES B type (35% of cases)	60%	(55% –68%)
DUKES C type (50% of cases)	30%	(25% –45%)

tumours than for higher lesions, whereas in some others (LOYGUE and DUBOIS 1966) the death rate is 4% after AP resection, 8% after anterior resection, and 6.5% after the Babcock operation.

General information drawn from the most recent series is reported in Table 1. Several criteria are analysed: the average rate is given with the extremes, lowest and highest, in brackets.

These figures summarize the present status of curative surgery, with an average cure rate of 50%. Lymphatic spread continues to be associated with a poor prognosis even after major excisional surgery.

b) Sequelae of Surgery

It is not proposed to detail all the complications which can occur after rectal excision. Some may follow any major abdominal operation, others are more specifically related to rectal surgery. The late complications following rectal excision are briefly summarized.

Retention of urine is common in male patients after AP resection and not exceptional after low anterior resection. Elderly patients with prostatic enlargement are especially prone to this complication, which is usually managed by transurethral resection. Urinary problems also occur in female patients after AP resection.

Disorders of sexual function in male patients are not uncommon. GOLIGHER (1977) says that "in younger patients this may on occasions prove a disastrous consequence of operation". In men over 60 the effect of surgery is less marked because a proportion already have some impairment of sexual activity. In women there may also be serious problems, although there is almost no mention of this complication in surgical reports.

In spite of the significant progress made during the past decade in helping patients towards a normal life by improving management of their colostomies and by the formation of colostomy care associations, the damaging psychological effect of a colostomy must not be underestimated. As GOLIGHER (1977) has stressed, for elderly patients in poor social conditions or patients living alone, a colostomy may become a major problem. Patients "feel isolated, depressed and lose all interest in feeding and looking after themselves". This situation may produce profound psychological upset and withdrawal, and can only be counteracted with help from those trained in the management of stomas and additional support from the community services.

3. Additional Therapy

Althouth there has been some progress in the 5-year survival rate of some reports of patients with curative surgery for cancer of the rectum, the overall general cure rate remains fairly constant at about 50%. When there is a gross involvement of the perirectal fat, or lymph node metastasis, the outlook for survival after curative resection is not better than 30%–40%. It seems unlikely that improvements in surgical technique will produce a significant increase in the number of patients who survive, unless early detection allows diagnosis at a more favourable stage of the disease.

Local recurrence is one of the principal causes of failure following surgery. After AP resection for cancer of the lower half of the rectum, most recurrences occur in the perineum or pelvic region (GILCHRIST and DAVID 1947). These recurrences are due to the presence of viable neoplastic cells beyond the surgical field, or to the spillage or dissemination of cancer cells during manipulation of the tumour at the time of the operation.

GILBERTSEN (1960) studied 125 patients with carcinoma of the rectum who died following curative resection. He found that 37% of these patients had evidence of local recurrence. CASS et al. (1976) analysed 280 patients who underwent a complete resection for cancer of the colon and rectum. Total local recurrence rate was 28%. Sixty-three patients had local recurrence alone, 15 had both local and distant tumours. The highest recurrence rates were in cases of poorly differentiated tumours and those extending through the bowel wall. GUNDERSON and SOSIN (1974) evaluated experience with second-look operations following curative resection in 75 patients with tumours extending beyond the bowel wall and/or in lymph nodes. Fifty-two (70%) had residual tumour at reoperation. Forty-eight (64%) had local or regional failures as a component of failure.

MORSON et al. (1963) found a 10% incidence of pelvic recurrence after excision for cancer of the rectum. They suggest that if all B and C DUKES tumours were submitted to post-operative irradiation, 85% of pelvic recurrences would be prevented. This would involve 58% of all patients in their series. REE et al. (1975) reported a 24% incidence of local recurrence in patients having undergone AP resection. The most recent data from the Massachusetts General Hospital indicate a local-regional recurrence rate of 29% in cases of macroscopic transmural tumour with negative lymph nodes, and a recurrence rate of 45% in the presence of macroscopic transmural tumours with positive lymph nodes (COHEN et al. 1981). The differences in the incidence of local recurrence according to these statistics are probably related to the criteria used to assess the relapses.

The use of radiotherapy as an adjuvant to surgery aims to decrease the rate of pelvic and perineal recurrence after radical excision of the rectum. Numerous trials, some randomized, using pre- or post-operative adjuvant therapy have been published during the past 10 years.

a) Pre-operative Irradiation

The rationale of pre-operative irradiation is to try to reduce viability of the tumour cells at operation by destroying, or rendering incapable of further growth, cancer cells already present in lymph nodes or perirectal tissues, and in this way reducing the incidence of recurrences due to seeding of malignant cells.

It has been suggested the pre-operative irradiation may achieve the objective of the so-called no-touch isolation technique popularized by TURNBULL (1974,

1975), which proved to be effective in limiting the spread of cancer cells in the surgical treatment of tumours of the large bowel situated above the level of the peritoneal reflexion.

After publication of a retrospective study at Memorial Sloan Kettering Cancer Center by STEARNS et al. (1959) much interest was aroused in the possible beneficial effects of pre-operative irradiation for patients with large tumours. The results of several studies, including a number of randomized or non-randomized trials, regarding the value of pre-operative radiotherapy have recently been published. Different protocols or irradiation have been suggested. They differ markedly as to target volume, total tumour dose, dose-time factor, and the optimum time interval between the completion of pre-operative radiation therapy and surgery.

The Veterans Administration Oncology Group conducted a prospective randomized study of 700 male patients presenting with operable rectal carcinoma. The results have been reported by HIGGINS (1972, 1979) HIGGINS and ROSWIT, HIGGINS et al. (1973), ROSWIT (1981) and HIGGINS et al. (1975). The patients were treated either by surgery alone or by radiotherapy prior to surgery. Radiotherapy was administrated in a dosage of 2000 rad over a 2-week period, with 500-rad boosters for those whose tumour was within 8 cm of the anal verge. Resection was carried out as soon as was feasible afterwards. The overall 5-year survival was 35% in the radiotherapy group, and 29% in those treated by surgery alone. The most substantial treatment benefit occurred with the combined therapy in patients with low-lying lesions undergoing curative AP resection. In the group of 305 patients divided into two equal subgroups, the 5-year survival rate was 47% in the treated group versus 34% in the surgical group.

Positive lymph nodes were found in only 27.8% in the combined therapy group versus 41.2% in the surgical group, with the largest difference being in those patients with low-lying tumours requiring AP resection (26% versus 44%). Local and regional recurrences were reduced (29% versus 40%). Pre-operative irradiation in no way hampered the surgery and did not induce complications. Autopsies demonstrated that residual tumour was present in 49% of the patients treated by radiotherapy and surgery, versus 68% in the surgical group.

A second pre-operative radiotherapy trial has been conducted by HIGGINS and ROSWIT (1981) since 1976. Only patients with rectal carcinoma at a level requiring AP resection as determined by clinical examination were included. The radiotherapy dosage was 3150 rad in 18 fractions of 175 rad over a 24-day period. Over 300 patients have been included in this trial, which is still in progress. Preliminary results based on 189 patients having undergone curative resection (primary tumour removed and no evidence of residual disease) showed improved 5-year survival in those patients given the combined therapy (60% versus 53%). HIGGINS (1981) emphasized that the survival advantage of treated patients in both trials occurs during the 3rd and 4th years, and that preliminary data suggest that the treatment benefit apparent in the first trial will be even more substantial in the second trial.

The non-randomized study begun in 1960 at the University of Oregon by STEVENS, ALLEN, and FLETCHER (1977) deserves a special mention. During a period of 12 years 104 patients were treated, 58 of whom were considered to have resectable tumours and 46 inoperable lesions before irradiation. A dose of 5000 rad was delivered to the area of the tumour over a 5–8 week period, with a 2-MeV photon beam or cobald-60. Surgical excision of the tumour occurred 4–7 weeks following the completion of irradiation.

Forty-four of the 58 patients with initially clinically resectable tumours had a subsequent curative resection, seven had a non-curative resection, and seven had no resection of the tumour. Of the 44 patients with curative resection, 24 (55%) were alive and free of tumour at 5 years. This rate is compared with the 38% 5-year tumour-free survival in patients with curative resection treated with surgery at the same institution. The results of pre-operative irradiation in this series are quite remarkable, considering that most patients were thought to have advanced disease originally. Positive nodes were found in 20% of the specimens. No tumour could be found in five specimens and only microfocal cancer was detected in an additional group of three patients. Among the patients who died, no local recurrence was found in the pelvis.

Seventeen of the 46 patients with initially clinically unresectable tumours had resection of the tumour within 10 weeks of completion of irradiation; two of them were alive and well at 5 and 10 years. Two patients died without tumour at 14 and 19 months. Tumour was totally sterilized by irradiation in nine patients, and reduced to a microfocal extent in an additional three of the total pre-operative group of 104 patients.

KLIGERMAN (1975, 1977), at the Yale New Haven Hospital, reported randomized series of 41 cases with a 5-year survival of 41% in the combined treatment group, compared with 25% in the surgical group. SIMBERTSEVA et al. (1975) from Leningrad published their experience of 242 patients treated either by surgery alone or by 3000 rad 1 week prior to surgery. The 6-year survival rates were respectively 40% for the patients treated by surgery, and 52.5% for patients who underwent pre-operative irradiation. They ascribed the significant reduction in local recurrence to the use of radiation.

GARY-BOBO et al. (1979; Montpellier, France), in a non-randomized study of combined radiosurgical treatment of rectal carcinoma, have treated 116 patients by means of surgical excision of rectal tumours after concentrated pre-operative irradiation, giving 4000 rad to the pelvic tumour volume in 18 sessions over 21 days. The operation consisted of AP excision in 79 cases and of anterior resection in 37 cases. The operation was carried out a few days after the completion of irradiation. The operative mortality was 7.7% and the complications due to radiotherapy itself were mainly a delay of perineal wound healing. Survival rate at 5 years was 59.5%. In 17 cases the surgery was only palliative because of unresectable tumours or liver metastasis. The node involvement noticed on the operative specimen was only 16.4%. If one considers only the cases treated with a curative purpose, the 5-year survival rate was 70%.

BUGAT et al. (1981) reported on a series of 96 patients with carcinoma of the rectum treated by preoperative irradiation at the Centre REGAUD, Toulouse, France, between 1976 and 1979. A dose of 3600 rad was delivered to the pelvis and the perineum by AP-PA portals in 15 fractions over 4 weeks. Surgery, usually AP resection, was performed 2 weeks after completion of irradiation. Surgery was considered curative in 75 cases. In three cases there was no more tumour in the operative specimen. The actuarial 2-year and 5-year survival rates were 94% and 70% respectively in the group of patients treated curatively.

Special experience of pre-operative irradiation was gained at the Mayo Clinic in the period 1914–1943, and published in 1961 by RUFF et al. Ninety-six patients were treated with radium and underwent excision 6 weeks later. The 5-year survival rate was 43.7%. The pathological changes have been carefully studied in operative specimens. It was demonstrated that radium can, at times, completely destroy an adenocarcinoma of the rectum. In ten cases no residual carcinoma was found in the operative specimen, but in most cases the lack of homogeneity of radium applied to large tumours has been confirmed by necrotic and actively growing tumour tissue seen side by side in the same microscopic section. However, radium made an inoperable lesion operable in ten cases, in four of which a 5-year survival was achieved.

From 1974 until 1978 the British Medical Research Council conducted a trial of pre-operative radiotherapy for rectal carcinoma. Seven hundred and eighty-four patients treated in various centres in Britain were included in a random study with three treatment options: a 2000-rad dosage given over a period of 10 days (multiple fraction group), a single dosage of 500 rad (single fraction group), and a control group (surgery alone). Surgery followed as soon as possible, preferably within 24 h of the radiation. Preliminary conclusions from the study reported by SMITH (1980) are that radiotherapy with a dose of 2000 rad significantly affects tumour size and tumour staging (fewer stage C than in the control group), but the long-term results have not yet been published. It was noticed that the single dose of 500 rad does not result in any change of tumour size and tumour staging.

RIDER (1975) reported on an randomized trial giving 500 rad to the tumour prior to surgery, compared to surgery alone. He found an improved crude 5-year survival (35% versus 19%) in those having received pre-operative radiotherapy.

If all the series are considered, the effects of pre-operative irradiation may be summarized as follows:
1. Reduction in size of bulky lesions and reduction in adherence to adjacent structures which may make the operation easier
2. Decrease in the expected rate of lymphatic involvement
3. Decrease in the rate of local recurrences
4. Increase in the survival rate.

Three questions remain:
1. How is one best to select the patients who will benefit from combined therapy?
2. What is the best protocol of irradiation?
3. What is the best time for surgery after irradiation?

Selection of Patients. Patients suitable for pre-operative irradiation are those who are most likely to develop local-regional recurrence after AP resection. There are operable patients with quite good expectation of life after surgery, who have extensive but resectable tumours of the lower two-thirds of the rectum. There are tumours largern than 5 cm in diameter, ulcerative and infiltrating, more or less stenosing, and with fair or impaired mobility. Consistency and mobility are good indicators of the transmural tumour penetration and of the risk of local recur-

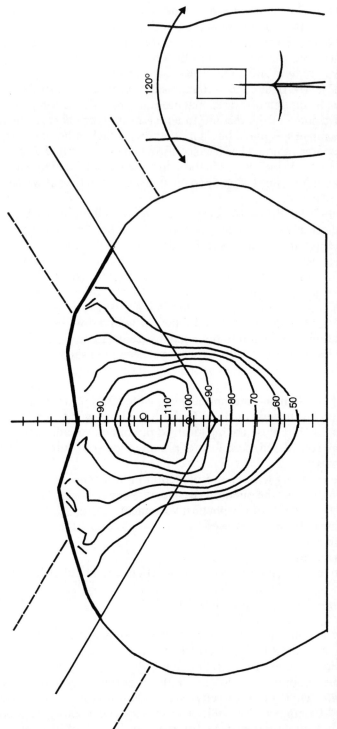

Fig. 3. Isodose distribution of pre-operative irradiation by Cobalt-60 for cancer of the middle third of the rectum, lower end of the tumour more than 7 cm above the anal verge, patient in prone position. Sacral field 10 × 14 cm, cobalt-60 arc therapy 120°. The axis of rotation is 10 cm depth. A dose of 3 000 rad calculated at 8 cm depth is delivered in ten fractions within 12 days

rence after curative surgery. In this group are included lesions which are perfectly resectable and marginally operable.

Lesions of the upper third of the rectum suitable for restorative procedures are not excluded from this pre-operative treatment, but they are best treated with post-operative radiation therapy of indicated according to the pathological criteria.

Excluded are: patients older than 75 years of age or in poor general condition; patients with fixed or disseminated lesions only amenable to palliation; patients with symptoms of bowel obstruction (because they are in need of immediate colostomy); patients with limited, freely mobile tumours easily curable by surgery alone (these can be submitted to combined treatment but do not present the best indications for pre-operative irradiation); patients with elevated plasma CEA level considered as having a likely disseminated disease.

A second group of patients with fixed, clinically unresectable tumours may be irradiated, but the purpose of irradiation in this case is to try to make the tumour operable and to give the patients some chance of control of their disease. In this field EMANI et al. (1979) treated 44 patients with unresectable cancer by irradiation at a dose of 4500–5000 rad. Twenty-six of the 44 cases were resected (70%) and 18 of 26 (70%) are alive and well more than 36 months later.

Definition of Protocol. A reliable protocol of irradiation should be simple and safe, with little morbidity. The dose of radiation must not be too high and the target volume should not include the para-aortic area. It should be limited to the pelvic area.

Two protocols of pre-operative irradiation are used at the Centre Léon Bérard. (a) When the tumour is more than 7 cm from the anal verge, irradiation is directed to the posterior part of the pelvis exclusively (Fig. 3). A tumour dose of 3000 rad is delivered in 10 fractions within 12 days by arctherapy, cobalt 60, or 18-MeV photons. The dose is calculated at 8 cm depth. A sacral field (10 × 14 cm) is used. The lower margin of the field is 3 cm above the anal orifice, the patient being in the prone position. (b) When the tumour is less than 7 cm from the anal verge, the target volume encompasses the posterior part of the pelvis and the anal area. A tumour dose of 3000 rad is delivered in ten fractions over 12 days. Two fields are used: through a perineal field a dose of 1500 rad calculated at 6 cm depth is delivered; and through a sacral field with a 45° wedge filter a dose of 1500 rad calculated at 8 cm depth is given. The dose at the surface of the perineum does not exceed 2200 rad (Fig. 4).

The tolerance is excellent. The operation takes place 4 or 5 weeks after completion of irradiation and there is no delay in the perineal wound healing attributable to radiotherapy.

Delay Between Radiotherapy and Surgery. In many surgical centres the radical excision is performed a few days after completion of the irradiation, whereas in others a free interval of 4–6 weeks exists between irradiation and surgery.

In pre-operative irradiation of breast cancer or uterine cervix carcinoma, the operation is never performed immediately after the last application of irradiation but usually 4–5 weeks later. There is no reason why this guideline should not be

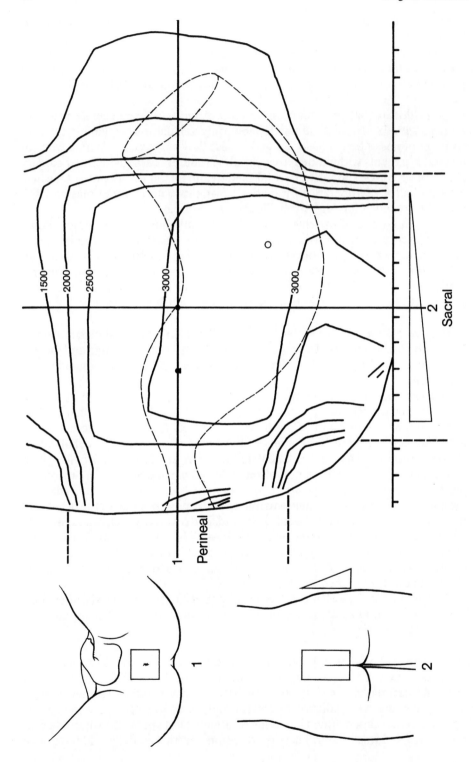

Additional Therapy

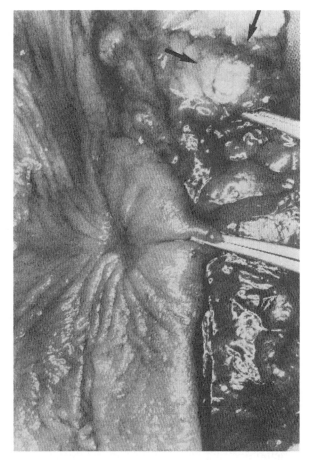

Fig. 5. Operative specimen of an AP resection performed 6 weeks after pre-operative irradiation (arc-therapy, Cobalt 3 000 rads in 12 days) for a patient with an ulcerative well-differentiated adenocarcinoma, 3 cm in diameter, located in the middle rectum with a metastatic lymph node palpable 2 cm above the primary tumor. There was no active tumor in the specimen. The primary tumor was locally controlled and replaced by a shallow ulcer. The node was necrotic without neoplastic cells *(arrow)*. No other metastatic nodes in the specimen.

applied in the case of rectal cancer. The post-operative morbidity is not increased when the AP resection or anterior resection is carried out 4–5 weeks after irradiation (Fig. 5). The only problem is psychological, since some patients may be reluctant to undergo major surgery after the relief of symptoms such as bleeding, discharge, or tenesmus by irradiation. This problem should not be underestimated and should be a matter of trust between the patient and the clinician.

Fig. 4. Technique of pre-operative irradiation by cobalt-60 for cancer of the lower third of the rectum. A dose of 3 000 rad is delivered in ten fractions over 12 days through two fields: a perineal field *(1)* 8 × 8 cm, and a sacral field *(2)* 8 × 10 cm with 45° wedge filter. The lower end of the perineal field is 3 cm above the anal verge. The maximum dose given to the perineum is 2 200 rad

The delay between irradiation and surgery is useful because the optimal biological effect of radiotherapy is only obtained after 4–5 weeks. The clinician is unable to foresee the radiosensitivity and the changes in the tumour which will occur during the weeks following irradiation. If in some cases there is only little change, in other cases the lesion will have shrunk a lot; its mobility and its size will be substantially improved. This can only be observed if operation does not take place immediately after irradiation (Fig. 5).

Critics of this combined therapy are concerned with three things:
1. The change in the tumour staging category and the difficulty for the pathologist in defining the histological grading of the carcinoma. It is true that major changes in the histological appearance of tumours are induced by irradiation, and that operative specimens after irradiation cannot be compared with specimens after surgery alone. The purpose of this combined treatment is to try to improve the cure rate, and these changes are a measure of the effectiveness of radiation therapy.
2. The possibility of post-operative complications, such as delayed perineal wound healing. As long as the irradiation is properly applied, at a reasonable dose on a target-volume limited to the perirectal area, there should not be an increased incidence of post-operative complications.
3. The psychological problems for the patient submitted to a prolonged course of treatment. As has been previously emphasized, it requires a good psychological balance on the part of the patient and a satisfactory understanding by the patient of the necessity of completing the two stages of treatment.

b) Pre-operative Chemotherapy and Radiotherapy Combined

Chemotherapy given alone has not increased the 5-year survival rate after radical surgery (MOERTEL 1975). In 1981, CARTER mentioned that "at this point, adjuvant chemotherapy cannot be recommended as routine treatment for curative resection for patients with large bowel cancer with a high potential for metastatic relapse. Although 5-FU has been extensively evaluated, it has made no significant impact on survival". By contrast, recent papers have raised the possibility of giving chemotherapy with radiation in the pre-operative treatment of rectal cancer. The most commonly used drugs are 5-Fluorouracil (5-FU) and Mitomycin C (MTC). BUROKER et al. (1976) and SISCHY et al. (1980) have reported on this combined treatment and have demonstrated that chemotherapy reinforces the effectiveness of radiation therapy.

Chemotherapy and radiotherapy are both started on day 1. The 5-FU is given in a dosage of 600 mg/m^2/24 h by a continuous infusion in dextrose solution via an intravenous catheter for four days. Mitomycin C is given as a bolus intravenous injection at a dose of 10–12 mg/m^2 on day 1 only. The irradiation is carried out at the same dosage and with the same fractionation as previously described. This combined regime is generally tolerated well. Major falls in the white cell count are rarely observed. Transient diarrhoea is the usual symptom and is controlled without difficulty.

Since 1972, BOULIS-WASSIF and HOP (1980) at the Rotterdamsch-Radiotherapeutisch Institut have conducted a randomized trial for patients with potentially resectable rectal cancer. The patients were selected at random for treatment in three groups: S, surgery alone; R, pre-operative irradiation; and C, pre-operative combined radiotherapy and 5-FU (375 mg/m^2/day for the first 4 days of irradiation). Radiotherapy consisted of delivering a dose of 3450 rad in 15 fractions over 18 days to a diamond and chimney field, with upper border at L$_2$ level, followed by surgery within 2 weeks. One hundred and forty-three patients entered into this trial. The corrected survival rate vor T$_3$ and T$_4$ categories showed statistically significant improvement in patients treated pre-operatively, and especially in the group of patients who received combined radiotherapy and 5-FU ($p < 0.01$). The authors concluded that despite the meagre number of patients included in this study, this form of combination therapy is decidedly superior to a single-mode treatment of rectal cancer.

In conclusion, it can be said that pre-operative radiotherapy, with or without a short course of chemotherapy (5-FU, MTC) increases the 5-year survival rate in certain patients with advanced but operable rectal cancer, without giving rise to significant additional morbidity. The use of chemotherapy has not altered the protocol of radiotherapy. Irradiation can be performed at the same dosage and with the same fractionation as usual.

c) Post-operative Irradiation

Several recent reports have stimulated interest in irradiation carried out after radical excision of rectal tumours. The advantages of post-operative irradiation over pre-operative irradiation are: (a) selection of cases suitable for irradiation, (b) operative assessment of the extent of the disease, (c) easy pathological study and grading of the tumour, and (d) better definition of the target volume. GUNDERSON and SOSIN (1974) and GUNDERSON et al. (1976) have evaluated 44 patients who were felt to run a high risk of local recurrence, and who were receiving post-operative irradiation (4500–6000 rad in 5–7 weeks). Their preliminary results report a low rate of failures within the irradiated field.

ROMSDAHL and WITHERS (1977, 1978) have used post-operative irradiation in non-randomized studies at the M.D. Anderson Hospital, Houston. A dose of 4500–5000 rad is given over 6 weeks after radical excision or anterior resection for tumours penetrating the entire bowel wall, or with regionally involved lymph nodes. The series of ROMSDAHL (1977) was updated by WITHERS et al. in 1979. Since 1972, more than 100 patients had been treated with therapy after apparently complete surgical resection. The results of adjuvant radiotherapy were compared to those obtained by surgery alone in an historical and concurrent series. Local control was significantly improved in all stages of the disease but there was no significant improvement in the rate or duration of survival except in those patients in whom the tumour had invaded adjacent pelvic organs. Major complications associated with adjuvant radiotherapy were radiation enteritis and small-bowel dysfunction, including eight obstructions requiring reoperation, with one death resulting.

ZUCALI et al. (1980), of the National Cancer Institute of Milan, have published an enthusiastic report of 21 cases (20 adenocarcinomas, one squamous cell carcinoma) treated by surgery (Miles' operations in 18 cases, anterior resection in three cases) and post-operative irradiation. The pelvis received a medium dose of 4500 rad over 5–7 weeks through AP, PA opposed fields. Six patients received a boost of 1000 rad on the perineum. Median follow-up after surgery was 33 months (range 24–63 months). Only one patient (5%) had a pelvic recurrence at the perineum. This figure is compared with the 40% rate of regional recurrences expected in "locally advanced" rectal and rectosigmoid cancers. It may be mentioned that not all tumours included in this series were locally advanced, since regional lymph node metastases were demonstrated in nine cases (43% of cases), and in seven cases the tumour was confined to the bowel wall. The median follow-up of 33 months is not long enough to assess in a non-randomized trial the definitive efficacy of post-operative irradiation, because pelvic recurrences can be postponed by radiation therapy. TURNER, et al (1977) GHOSSEIN et al. (1981) reported on a series of 125 patients treated by post-operative irradiation after surgery for colorectal cancer. The average follow-up was 38 months, minimum 12 months, maximum 84 months. Of the 78 patients with rectosigmoid cancer 67% were alive and free of disease. The percentage of patients alive and well was the same in cases of complete resection of cancer or of microscopic residual disease. It was only half as much in cases of gross residual cancer after surgery.

Several other trials are in progress. Those of the GITSG and Radiation Therapy Oncolocy Group (RTOG) deserve special mention.

Objectives of the study conducted by the GITSG were to compare the effects of post-operative radiotherapy with and without adjuvant chemotherapy and with chemotherapy alone on duration of disease-free interval, local recurrence rates, and overall survival in patients who had undergone curative surgery for rectal carcinoma. Entry was limited to rectal adenocarcinomas stage Dukes B and C. The distal edge of the primary had to be no more than 12 cm from the anal verge.

Patients in the radiotherapy-only arm received 4000 or 4800 rad total dose given over 4.5–5.5 weeks. The dosage schedule in the chemotherapy-only arm was: 5-FU, 325 mg/m^2/day IV on days 1–5; Me-CCNU, 130 mg/m^2 orally on day 1. This course of chemotherapy was repeated every 10 weeks for 18 months. The combination arm schedule was: radiotherapy 4000–4400 rad total dose given over 4.5–5.5 weeks; chemotherapy: 5-FU 500 mg/m^2/day IV on the first 3 and last 3 days of radiotherapy; beginning 5 weeks later, 5-FU 300 mg/m^2/day IV for 5 days plus Me-CCNU 100 mg/m^2/day orally once; 10 days later, 5-FU 375 mg/m^2/day IV for 5 days. Fifteen weeks later, chemotherapy was resumed as in the the chemotherapy-only arm and continued for 18 months.

Two-year results of this trial show a decrease in recurrence rates for the combined modality compared with surgery-only controls. The study was activated in 1975. With median follow-up of 118 weeks, recurrence rates were:
Surgery only (either AP or anterior resection), 52%
Radiotherapy only, 32%
Chemotherapy (5-FU and Me-CCNU) only, 39%
Combined chemotherapy and radiotherapy, 21%.

The difference between the surgery-only control group and the other three arms was statistically significant ($p = 0.05$). The difference between the surgery group and the radiotherapy-chemotherapy arm was very significant ($p = 0.001$).

Local recurrence rates demonstrated less significant differences, except for the combined modality rate: 19% for surgery only; 15% for radiotherapy only; 23% for chemotherapy only; and 3% for radiotherapy and chemotherapy combined. The improvements for the adjuvant therapy arms seemed so striking that the GITSG terminated patient entry into the surgery-only arm in February 1980.

However CARTER (1981) warned against placing too much emphasis on the 2-year results, insisting that 2 more years of follow-up were needed to determine whether the improvement in the adjuvant arms will hold up.

A protocol including both pre- and post-operative radiotherapy the "sandwich" technique) is at present being conducted by the RTOG. It consists of:
1. A randomization between surgery alone and pre-operative irradiation (500 rad to the tumoural area 24 h prior to surgery).
2. Post-operative pathological staging, which distinguishes between patients with DUKES' A tumour, who do not receive any further treatment, and patients with DUKES' B or C tumour.
3. Post-operative irradiation for patients with DUKES' B or C tumour at a dosage of 4500 rad over 5–6 weeks, to a target volume which extends from a upper margin at L_5–S_1 to the perineum. Irradiation is performed through AP/PA fields plus lateral fields.

Every effort is advised to reduce the amount of small bowel in the treatment field, using, for instance, a compression device over the anterior pelvis or using only a posterior and two lateral fields. Stress is also placed on the danger of severe radiation reaction in the perineal folds in both sexes by utilization of opposed AP/PA portals for the entire course of treatment.

MOHUIDDIN et al. (1981) reported a series of 62 patients treated with "selective sandwich" adjuvant radiotherapy in a pilot study which began in 1976. All patients received the single pre-operative dose of 500 rads. Forty-four patients underwent AP resection, four patients a low anterior resection, ten patients a combined abdominotranssacral resection, and four found to have liver metastasis had colostomy followed by palliative therapy. Twenty-one patients (Dukes A) were given no further therapy. Of 37 patients with stage B or C, 21 received postoperative irradiation. Follow-up ranges from 6 to 36 months with a median of 18 months. Two of 21 patients receiving post-operative irradiation have developed metastatic disease; neither has failed in the pelvis. Of 16 patients who did not receive post-operative irradiation, three have had metastasis to the pelvis and two others have developed distant metastasis. The authors concluded that this approach warrants investigation for its potential efficacy in randomized studies such as that undertaken by the RTOG.

Technique of Post-operative Irradiation. From a technical point of view, some arrangements of fields protect the small bowel and prevent prohibitive reaction of the perineal area, while delivering a high and homogeneous dose of radiation to the target volume. In this regard the irradiation applied according to the protocol used at the Centre Léon Bérard, Lyon is particularly well tolerated. Post-opera-

Surgical Treatment

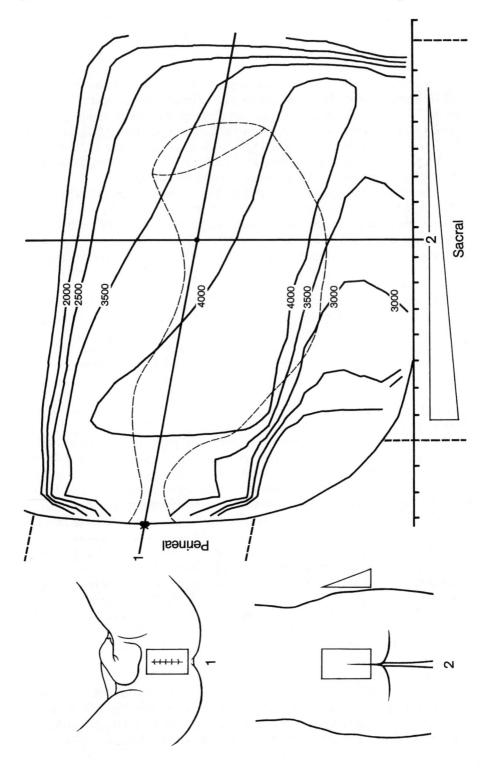

tive irradiation following AP resection is performed through two fields (perineal and sacral) with cobalt-60 (Fig. 6). The aim is to deliver a dose of 3 500 rad over 19 days to a target volume encompassing the perineal area and the presacral area, with a satisfactory protection of the small bowel and urinary bladder. Two fields are used: through a perineal field a given dose of 3 600 rad (at the surface) is delivered in nine fractions (the beam is inclined 10° downwards on the horizontal line). Through a sacral field a dose of 2 000 rad is delivered in six fractions with a 45° wedge filter. The isodose curve shows that an homogeneous dose is delivered to the whole target volume and only a small dose to the small bowel in the pelvis. The tolerance is quite good.

After anterior resection in cases of tumour of the upper third of the rectum which has invaded the perirectal fat or serosa, post-operative irradiation using cobalt-60 in arc-therapy of 120° is justified. The protocol consists of delivering a dose of 3 000 rad in ten fractions over 16 days through a sacral field measuring 7 × 12 cm. The axis of rotation is 10 cm deep and the dose is calculated at 8 cm. The target volume is centred by the area of the rectocolic anastomosis. Before starting treatment it is advisable to carry out a barium examination of the small bowel to gain some idea of the location of the small intestine in the Douglas pouch in its relation to the irradiated area, and to adapt the technique so that only a limited part of the small bowel is irradiated.

It is not possible at present to reconcile protagonists of pre-operative and post-operative irradiation as additive therapies to surgery for rectal cancer. Both have advantages and disadvantages.

Pre-operative irradiation applied to cases suitable for such combined therapy has proved to be effective in increasing the cure rate, without inducing major morbidity. But this method requires collaboration between surgeon and radiotherapist. The decision to use irradiation depends on the surgeon referring the patient to the radiotherapist.

Post-operative irradiation affords the advantage of knowledge of the extent of tumour at surgery; the radiation can be given to those at greatest risk of recurrence, i.e. with tumours which have spread through the bowel wall or into adjacent structures and/or with positive lymph nodes. However, pretreatment evaluation, especially the histological differentiation, consistency, and mobility of the tumour, give quite a clear idea of the extent of the tumour and of the probability of recurrence after surgery.

The site of the tumour in the rectum may be useful in the choice between pre- or post-operative irradiation. For tumours located in the upper third of the rectum there may be fewer problems with anterior resection combined with post-operative irradiation than in pre-operatively irradiated patients. But post-operative irradiation has the disadvantages of not affecting cells which may spread at the

Fig. 6. Post-operative irradiation by Cobalt-60 following AP resection. A dose of 3 500 rad is delivered to the target volume in 15 fractions over 19 days. Two fields are used. Through a perineal field *(1)* 8 × 8 cm a given dose of 3 600 rad is delivered in nine fractions of 400 rad. Through a sacral field *(2)* 8 × 15 cm, a dose of 2 000 rad calculated at 8 cm depth is delivered with a 45° wedge filter, in six fractions. Protection of the anterior part of the pelvis and small bowel is satisfactory

time of surgery, giving no improvement in resectability and causing, small-bowel complications if the bowel is fixed with adhesions following surgery when the target volume is extensive. Sometimes, due to late perineal wound healing, postoperative irradiation is started only 3 months after surgery. In any case radiation should be limited to the pelvic area or part of the pelvis, and the dose should not exceed 4500 rad in 5 weeks if severe side-effects are to be avoided. So far it is impossible to evaluate the advantages of post-operative irradiation. For this reason we prefer the pre-operative irradiation. It has proved to be efficient in decreasing the rate of local recurrence for locally advanced extramural tumours of the lower two-thirds of the rectum.

A particular case is represented by elderly and frail patients with rather large but not too infiltrating tumor suitable for APR. Preoperative irradiation may reduce the size of the lesion in such a manner that it becomes suitable for conservative procedure. Thanks to the delay (6–8 weeks) after preoperative irradiation patients are given a chance of sphincter preservation.

IV. Rationale of Conservative Treatment for Cure

In 1974, TURNBULL wrote that "a new era was dawning for rectal cancer, the era of small highly curable cancers". He pointed out that surgeons were seeing an increasing number of patients with very small mobile cancers, which "could be treated without recourse to radical surgery".

The objective of the local treatment of rectal cancer is ambitious. The patient must have a chance of cure equal to that following major surgery, but without wide excision, and especially without permanent colostomy. To speak of a purely local treatment for rectal cancer would have been considered a dangerous heresy some years ago, because this idea was diametrically opposed to the principles of cancer surgery held at that time.

During the past decade there have been significant changes of opinion, and although major surgery remains the conventional approach to rectal cancer, conservative procedures have gained a place in selected cases. In 1974, BEAHRS noted that "the surgeon in dealing with cancer of the rectum, should leave his options open, and, considering all factors regarding the particular lesion, the health and welfare of the patient, make a judgement that will offer the patient the best chance of cure and satisfactory quality of life thereafter." He added that *"the theoretical advantage of radical surgery may be offset by the mortality of the procedure and if lesions are carefully selected for a conservative procedure, the survival rate compares favorably or is better than when radical surgery is used."*

Several factors have contributed to this change. Professional and educational programmes with their publicity, the increase in the number of patients screened by complete physical examination including rectal investigation, and more frequent use of the Haemocult test have all helped towards the earlier diagnosis of rectal cancer. During the same period a better understanding of the pathology of the early stages of the disease has evolved. Finally, an increasing awareness of the inconvenience of permanent colostomy has persuaded surgeons to try to preserve normal anal function, without jeopardizing the chance of cure.

Three conditions must be fulfilled before conservative treatment is proposed: (a) strict selection of cases, (b) proper schedules for treatment, and (c) regular follow-up of the patient after treatment. These rules must be followed exactly. Any attempt to overstep the limits of the indications for conservative treatment will jeopardize the survival of patients who would be cured by radical surgery. Control of the tumour will be obtained only if the correct technique is used. Each method requires care and experience, for any failure will discredit the method. Lastly, conservative procedures are only applicable to patients who are available to be followed up regularly for many years. Conservative treatment of limited rectal cancer makes considerable demands on the attending physician or surgeon as well as the patient, and must not be regarded lightly.

1. Selection of Suitable Cases

After local treatment for cure there is no mortality, there should be little or no morbidity, and sphincter function should be entirely normal. The selection of cases suitable for such treatment depends on three factors: (a) the risk of lymphatic spread, (b) the site of the tumour, and (c) the status of the patient.

a) Risk of Lymphatic Spread

One of the main arguments in favour of major surgery is the need to remove the regional lymph nodes. The rationale for radical surgery is based on three assumptions:
1. All invasive rectal carcinomas, whatever their size, can give rise to lymphatic spread.
2. The risk of nodal involvement in each individual is unpredictable.
3. Metastatic nodes cannot be detected clinically.

It is true that all invasive rectal carcinomas may involve the lymphatics, but the probability of nodal involvement depends on the histological features and the extent of the tumour. Although lymphangiography and the CAT scanner are unable to visualize the pelvic lymph nodes draining the rectum in the majority of cases, the clinician is not completely helpless in his search for pararectal metastatic nodes.

For a start, local treatments are directed at the rectal tumour alone; they are not concerned with the lymphatic chains. By definition, they are applied to only those cancers which are thought to have no lymphatic spread and therefore a high probability of being local disease confined to the rectum.

The risk of lymphatic involvement depends on three factors: (a) the degree of histological differentiation, (b) the local spread, and (c) the absence of palpable metastatic nodes in the pelvis.

Degree of Differentiation. Following studies of the histological features of tumours, particularly the grade of malignancy, it is possible to assess the risk of lymphatic spread in each individual case of rectal cancer. All poorly differentiated adenocarcinomas and colloid carcinomas, known for their high potential of dissemination, have to be excluded from conservative treatment. They are only suitable for the most radical procedures with poor chances of cure. Only well- or fairly well differentiated adenocarcinomas can be accepted in the framework of conservative measures. Multiple biopsies taken at several points of the tumour are required before deciding to start local therapy.

Local Spread. Lymphatic involvement is related to local spread. The assessment of the degree of infiltration of the rectal wall aims to identify the lesions penetrating through the rectal wall, which must be treated by radical procedures. Growths confined to the rectal wall which have a much lower probability of nodal involvement – 6% for polypoid cancers, 12% for ulcerative cancers – may be suitable for local treatment.

Until recently the classification of rectal tumours was based on pathological examination of the specimen obtained at operation. However, MASON (1976a) has proposed a clinical staging based on the mobility of the tumour determined by digital examination. The purpose of this classification, applicable only to tumours located in the lower half of the rectum, is to answer the question: "Can we hope to assess the extent of the disease, which could be helpful in the therapeutic procedure applied to each individual patient and especially to restorative or conservative treatment". MASON started by trying to correlate what he could determine before operation with what he could see in longitudinal macrosections cut through the fixed resected specimen. He has described four clinical stages (CSs):

CSI: The growth is freely mobile. It corresponds to a tumour in which the loose connective tissue space between the muscular mucosae and the muscle coat of the rectum has not as yet been involved.

CSII: The tumour is mobile, but the index finger can appreciate that the mobility is less than that of a CSI tumour. In such a case, the muscle coat has been invaded but the growth has not passed through it.

CSIII: The growth gives the examining finger the impression of a "tethered mobility". The growth and the wall move together. It is due to the penetration in the perirectal fatty tissue. Two degrees of extramural spread are noted: CSIII (−) or CSIII (+).

CSIV: The tumours, which have transgressed the pararectal space to invade an adjacent structure, may be fixed or have a tethered fixation due to adhesion either to the bone or to an organ which is mobile, such as uterus or posterior vaginal wall.

In fact, the clinician facing this problem is able to assess local spread quite accurately, basing his findings not only on the mobility, which is the most important sign of penetration of the bowel, but also on the appearance of the growth and on its consistency. Well-differentiated polypoid cancers, which are usually not very hard and freely mobile, are slightly infiltrating and always confined to the rectal wall. When there is a polypoid cancer beyond the reach of the index finger, between 9 cm and 12 cm above the anal verge, the clinical findings are not so accurate, but an impression of the consistency and mobility may be obtained with the tip of the rectoscope. Ulcerative well-differentiated adenocarcinomas represent the most difficult challenge. The degree of infiltration of the rectal wall can only be assessed if the tumour is within reach of the examining finger, i.e. in the distal 9 cm of the rectal ampulla. Ulcerative tumours always infiltrate the bowel to some extent; palpation shows that some growths are more indurated than others. A slough in the centre of an ulcer is often a sign of penetration of the perirectal tissue. It may not be easy to distinguish between true mobility (MASON's CSI) and tethered mobility (CSII and III).

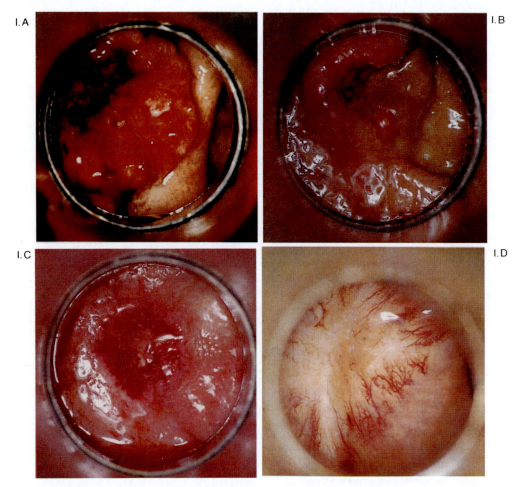

Plate 1. The "third week test" is used to assess the degree of infiltration of the rectal wall in case of ulcerative carcinoma

Fig. I. A. Ulcerative well differentiated adenocarcinoma (5 cm in diameter). Only one part of the tumor is visible in the lumen of the rectoscope, before treatment. (Contact + Iridium implant).

Fig. I. B. The same tumor three weeks later after two applications of Contact X-ray therapy (two overlapping fields). Significant shrinkage of the tumor (to only 2.5 cm in diameter). The ulceration has become shallow. The third week test proved that the tumor had no transmural penetration and was suitable for intracavitary irradiation.

Fig. I. C. Five weeks after the start of Contact X-ray therapy. All the exophytic part of the tumor has disappeared. Ulceration remains, with hardening of the rectal wall, necessitating interstitial curietherapy.

Fig. I. D. Final result after booster dose (2000 rads) given by interstitial curietherapy. A white scar with a crown of telangiectasia, but the rectal wall is really supple. The patient is well and disease-free after more than ten years.

Selection of Suitable Cases

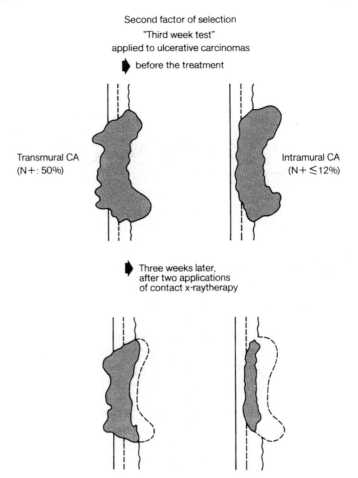

Fig. 7. Third week test. In the selection of ulcerative carcinomas the comparison of the tumour on the 1st day and on the 21st day after two applications of contact X-ray therapy is useful. Tumours with transmural penetration remain large and indurated and must be treated by radical surgery. Tumours confined to the bowel wall shrink a lot, and become smaller and less indurated. They can be accepted for curative intracavitary irradiation. $N+$, percentage of node involvement

In such cases, the radiotherapist has an additional means of assessment at his disposal. Contact X-ray therapy can be used to obtain a better idea of the degree of penetration of the rectal wall by the tumour.

Third Week Test. Two applications of contact X-ray therapy to the rectal lesion on days 1 and 8 allow the radiotherapist and the clinician to assess the degree of infiltration (Fig. 7). On the 21st day, 2 weeks after the second application of intracavitary irradiation, the response of the tumour to treatment is assessed. The shrinkage of some ulcerative cancers produces a complete change in their appearance. Their consistency is softer, their size has decreased, they are less infiltrating, more mobile, and the ulceration is not so deep. These changes prove that

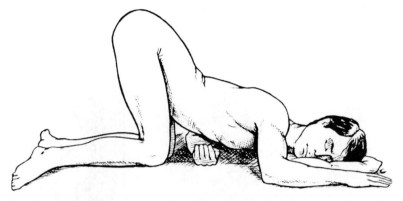

Fig. 8. Rectal examination performed with the patient in the knee-chest position allows an accurate assessment of the features of the tumour and a search for the pararectal metastatic nodes in cases of low-lying rectal cancer. Notice that the thighs are at 90° to the couch, the back hollowed, the head turned to the right, and the left forearm under the stomach

these tumours are confined to the bowel wall. Other tumours remain indurated, with a sloughing central crater, and the same impression of tethered mobility, which is a sign of penetration into the perirectal tissues. The former tumours are suitable for local and conservative therapy, the latter are only suitable for radical procedures and the patients must be referred to the surgeon immediately. The short delay of 3 weeks necessary to get a better appreciation of the local spread does not interfere with the prognosis of the rectal cancer in any way.

Absence of Palpable Metastatic Nodes in the Pelvis. GABRIEL et al. (1935) have demonstrated that the first lymph nodes to be involved by tumours are located in the mesorectum above the primary tumour, in its close vicinity, and that discontinuous lymphatic extension is very uncommon. If the growth is situated low in the rectum, it is possible to detect such metastatic nodes by a careful digital examination as long as this investigation is properly performed.

In most countries of the Western world, digital and endoscopic examination of the anorectal area are carried out with the patient lying in the left lateral position.

In France, however, digital examination is performed with the patient in the lithotomy position or the knee-chest position (Fig. 8). It is necessary to emphasize the great care that must be taken in rectal examination, and to point out the superiority of the knee-chest position for the detection of nodes in the mesorectum when compared with left lateral and lithotomy positions. The purpose of this examination is not only to assess the features of the rectal tumour, but also to palpate the rectal wall, especially above the rectal lesion, and to examine structures outside the rectum.

After appropriate preparation of the rectum, examination should involve three steps: A. palpation, endoscopy, and palpation. In female patients the digital examination includes a vaginal examination to supplement rectal palpation, particularly when the tumour is situated anteriorly, to determine if there is extension into the rectovaginal wall.

Selection of Suitable Cases

The patient is placed in the knee-chest position with the thighs at 90° to the couch, the back hollowed, the left arm under the stomach, the head turned to the right, lying directly on the couch. The position may be uncomfortable for elderly or obese patients, who must be supported. However, as MUIR (1960) has stated, this position permits the contents of the pelvis to fall upwards into the abdominal cavity and the walls of the rectum to fall apart, thus allowing a better assessment of the whole anorectal area and the lower part of the pelvic cavity. In contrast, in the left lateral or in the lithotomy position, the rectal lumen tends to collapse and the findings of digital and endoscopic examination are less accurate. These positions of the patient may be used secondarily. The first introduction of the index finger must be made slowly. Viscous Xylocaine lidocaine is helpful to reduce anal spasm and discomfort for the patient. The first palpation is used to gain an approximate idea of the features of the growth and as a preliminary to endoscopy. It is performed with the right or left index finger according to the site of the rectal lesion.

Rectoscopy is carried out, preferably with a wide tube 22–25 mm in diameter, in order to obtain a view in relief of the lesion and its surrounding mucosa, with the patient still in the knee-chest position. A fresh biopsy is taken. The second palpation summarizes and corroborates the impression given by the two previous steps of the examination. It aims especially to appreciate the consistency and mobility of the growth, its relation to extrarectal structures, and the presence or absence of metastatic nodes in the mesorectum above the primary tumour.

As has been noted by GOLIGHER (1977), "the extent to which the finger can be inserted into the rectum depends on the length of the operator's finger, and on the build of the patient and his willingness to relax his sphincter muscle". In most patients, and especially in females, by forcing the perineum upwards with the base of the finger, the range of palpation may be extended to about 10 cm above the anal verge. In stout men with heavy buttocks, digital penetration may only reach the distal 2–3 cm above the anal canal with difficulty. In such cases, general anaesthesia may be required to examine the lower half of the rectal ampulla adequately and make a decision about the use of conservative treatment.

A systematic search for metastatic nodes in the mesorectum is not commonly employed. When the growth is low, one can by careful palpation assess the suppleness of the rectal wall in each direction, anteriorly, posteriorly, and laterally, above the primary tumour with the patient in the knee-chest position. MUIR (1960) mentioned that "glands may be palpable in the mesorectum".

A metastatic pararectal lymph node is easily recognizable by its hardness, its shape (round or ovoid), its size (0.5–1.5 cm or more in diameter), and its mobility within the rectal wall. They are usually located on the same side of the rectum as the tumour. TURNBULL (1974) stated that "any hard, palpable nodule is a malignant node, with metastases in it. One does not feel inflammatory nodes that do not have cancer in them". He added that "it may be that there are some cancer cells here that may show up in later years and that a node will become palpable at follow-up examination after local therapy". Hypogastric nodes are less easily palpable. They are fixed to the lateral pelvic wall. This search for metastatic lymph nodes is a very useful way of approaching the problem of lymphatic dissemination when contemplating local treatment for tumours in the lower part of

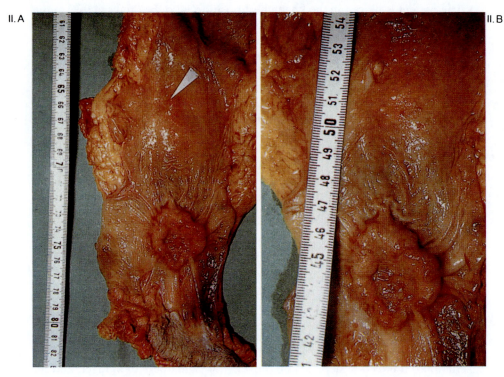

Plate 2

Fig. II. A. Operative specimen of a 50-year old female patient referred to the radiotherapist for intracavitary irradiation of this limited, ulcerative, well differentiated adenocarcinoma (2.8 cm on diameter). Rectal digital examination showed a small nodule in the meso-rectum. The patient was not irradiated and underwent an A. P. resection. The arrow shows the place of the hard nodule discovered by palpation.

Fig. II. B. The same specimen (close up) after incision of the mucosa. The metastatic nodule is visible (4 mm in diameter). No other metastatic lymh node.

the rectum. The presence of a node in the mesorectum is an indication for radical surgery.

The absence of indurated nodes in the rectal wall, in the first 3–4 cm above the rectal cancer, taken in conjunction with the histological features and the assessment of local spread, allows conservative treatment of these tumours to be undertaken in a controlled manner with relative safety.

In the series from the Centre Léon Bérard, metastatic nodes were found at the time of the initial assessment in 15 cases. Twelve patients were operated upon. The presence of metastatic nodes was confirmed in the operative specimen in 14 patients, and by the extension of the disease in the patient who was not operated upon. The search for metastatic nodes by palpation of the rectal wall above the site of the primary lesion must be performed systematically at each examination during the follow-up period. At the Centre Léon Bérard a suspicious node was found in 16 cases. All were treated surgically. Twelve of these nodes were malignant, and the patients underwent either a radical excision or a conservative procedure such a perirectal lymphadenectomy. The details of these cases will be given later. In four cases the nodule was benign: one patient underwent an AP resection, and the other three underwent local surgery.

The results of this search for metastatic nodes are shown in Table 2.

Table 2. Rectal adenocarcinoma: Search for palpable pararectal metastatic nodes[a]

No. of cases	Nodes found at the time of decision	Nodes found during the follow-up period
31	15 14 metastatic nodes 1 venous node of permeation	16 12 malignant lymph nodes 4 benign nodules (various origin)

[a] Centre Léon Bérard.

These results demonstrate the usefulness of the clinical search for metastatic nodes. Surprisingly, in most if not all reported series of local excision or electrocoagulation, except in that of TURNBULL (1974), no mention is made of the discovery of metastatic lymph nodes. This approach is mandatory whenever it is possible, before any decision is made regarding a local treatment and during the follow-up period.

Elective Inferior Mesenteric and Extra-mesenteric Lymphadenectomy for Rectal Cancer. It has often been said that the main objection to local treatment is the lack of knowledge of the presence or absence of lymph node metastases. It has been demonstrated that, in the case of a low-lying tumour, this approach to the assessment of the probability of lymphatic involvement is of value. However, there may be uncertainty about what is happening in the pelvis above the treated area after control of the primary tumour, especially when the lesion is located in the middle third of the rectum. In such cases the rectal wall above the treated area is not accessible to the examining finger. The problem of lymphatic dissemina-

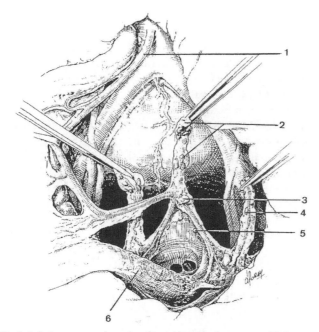

Fig. 9. Inferior mesenteric and perirectal lymphadenectomy. Main stage of the operation. *1*, Inferior mesenteric artery; *2*, paracolic glands; *3*, main superior haemorrhoidal lymph node; *4*, middle haemorrhoidal nodes; *5*, pararectal nodes; *6*, rectum.

tion is so important that when an ulcerative carcinoma has been locally controlled in a robust, middle-aged patient, an exploratory laparotomy with superior haemorrhoidal and perirectal lymphadenectomy may be proposed as a safety measure.

The purpose of the operation is to check the main lymphatic drainage areas of the rectum and to explore the pelvis, without bowel excision. This operation, which was initiated by MAYER et al. (1982) head of the Centre Léon Bérard, can be performed 2–3 months after completion of the conservative treatment by intracavitary irradiation.

The principle of the procedure may be criticized, and the treatment of lymphatics remote from the primary tumour may seem to be illogical for rectal cancer. However, in oncology this principle is commonly applied for epidermoid carcinomas of the mouth, lip, pharynx, or anal margin, and has proved to be effective. When the patient is a good surgical risk, under 55 years of age, with limited ulcerative well-differentiated carcinoma, laparotomy with lymphadenectomy is somewhat better than follow-up examination alone.

Inferior mesenteric and extra-mesenteric lymphadenectomy performed in such conditions may be considered an answer to the main objection to conservative treatment that does not involve the lymphatic drainage areas. For the radiotherapist it represents a form of collaboration with the surgeon. If no involved nodes are detected, the patient is followed up regularly; if metastatic nodes are found, radical surgery is immediately performed.

The technique of inferior mesenteric and extra-mesenteric lymphadenectomy for rectal cancer (Fig. 9) is as follows. Through a mid-line incision the liver is examined and the para-aortic and common external iliac nodes are palpated to check that the tumour has not spread throughout the abdomen. Then the sigmoid colon is freed from its congenital adhesions to the peritoneum in the left iliac fossa. Left and right ureters are identified at the level of the iliac arteries. The posterior parietal peritoneum is incised above and below the origin of the inferior mesenteric artery. The incision follows the right side of the rectum, and crosses in front of the rectum, entering the pouch of Douglas before continuing along the left side of the rectum up to the origins of the sigmoid arteries. Inferior mesenteric nodes are resected after the artery has been isolated at its origin. The dissection is extended along the artery up to the trunk of the sigmoid arteries. Sigmoid nodes are excised, and if there is any suspicion about their nature they are sent for a frozen section examination.

The dissection of the mesorectum is then undertaken. The operator enters the retrorectal space with his right hand. The posterior surface of the rectum is freed from the sacrum down to the levator ani muscles. Then the inferior mesenteric lymphadenectomy is performed with excision of all tissues bearing lymph nodes surrounding the artery. The lateral ligaments of the rectum are stretched and the superior haemorrhoidal pedicle is isolated at its origin and held in a ligature. With his left hand, the operator pulls this pedicle above and to the left, while the assistant, with his right hand, pushes the rectosigmoid colon anteriorly and to the left. A good exposure of the mesorectum is obtained. The bifurcation of the superior haemorrhoidal artery is identified and the principal nodes are excised and sent for frozen section. The dissection is continued successively along the right, and then the left branch of the superior haemorrhoidal artery up to their entry into the muscular layer of the rectal wall, and any lymphatic tissue is excised. This dissection, which exposes the posterior and lateral sides of the rectum with minimal blood loss, permits excision of the anorectal lymph nodes. Ligation of one of the branches of the superior haemorrhoidal artery may be necessary if its termination is surrounded by fibrotic tissue. Sometimes the nodes may be adherent to the rectal wall, which is repaired with silk thread. Then the middle haemorrhoidal pedicles are sectioned near their points of origin and tissues bearing lymph nodes are excised up to the rectal wall. The next stage of the operation is the excision of the posterior obturator lymph nodes situated at the bifurcation of the primitive iliac artery. A suction drain is put into the posterior rectal space and brought out through the left or right iliac fossa. The pelvic and parietal peritoneum is sutured and the abdomen is closed. After surgery recovery is rapid, and in the series at the Centre Léon Bérard no complications have been recorded.

b) Site of Tumour

When easily palpable tumours are located in the lower half of the rectum, conservative treatment may be considered as an alternative to treatment by radical excision and a permanent colostomy.

In general, when a cancer of the upper half of the rectum can be treated by anterior resection with restoration of intestinal continuity, conservative procedures have little place in its management. This concept is straightforward, and ulcerative lesions of the upper half of the rectum are treated by major surgery. Local treatment can be undertaken for freely mobile polypoid cancers between 9 cm and 12 cm from the anal verge, especially in poor-risk patients. In these circumstances the purpose of conservative measures is to avoid all types of major procedure, including restorative surgery.

The site of the tumour in the different segments of the lower rectum influences the choice of the method used for treatment. Tumours of the anterior wall of the rectum in female patients, tumours of the posterior wall more or less hidden in the concavity of the sacral bone, and tumours of the juxta-anal area invading the inner margin of the anal canal are treated in different ways. These procedures will be discussed in the chapter devoted to the comparison of the various methods of conservative treatment.

c) Status of Patient

More than one-fifth of all patients who present with cancer of the rectum may be considered as poor surgical risks. They form a large group of elderly (over 75 years of age), frail, senile patients with cardiovascular or respiratory problems, patients with cerebral insufficiency, extreme obesity, patients suffering from diabetes, or those who dread the prospect of a permanent colostomy. All these patients can be considered as borderline candidates for surgery. BEAHRS (1974) has emphasized that in these cases the added mortality and morbidity of radical surgery should be taken into consideration.

Age is obviously an important factor, and approximately two-thirds of the patients treated conservatively are elderly. In spite of the significant progress which has been made in pre- and post-operative medical care, improving the operability of elderly patients and decreasing the mortality rate significantly, it must be recalled that there are many problems among elderly patients. Some of them, who look younger than they really are and who seem in good general condition, will recover very well after major surgery; for some others the operation will have a prolonged effect on their physical and mental balance for the few years they have to live.

If one considers the mortality rate in elderly patients with „local" cancers of the lower half of the rectum on the one hand, and the risk of lymphatic spread and the chance of cure in cases of lymphatic involvement on the other hand, the survival figures are in the same range and usually favour conservative procedures. To illustrate this problem, STEARNS (1976) reported a series of 71 patients aged 70 or over who were treated by resection; six (8.3%) of them died after operation, and only four of 27 with regional nodal metastases were cured – a net loss of two patients.

It is now agreed that conservative treatment for limited rectal cancers may be regarded as an alternative to radical surgery, especially in patients over 75. These methods can also be applied to younger patients when the radiotherapist or the surgeon is especially aware of the limitations of local treatment.

2. Proper Schedules for Treatment

A successful outcome after conservative treatment implies not only the right choice of procedure but also expert application of that procedure. If poor judgement is combined with inadequate treatment, the survival of the patient will be jeopardized.

Conservative treatment may employ a number of surgical or radiotherapeutic techniques. Each method has its own effectiveness and its own indications, limitations, advantages, and complications. The clinician must select the patient with a tumour suitable for treatment by conservative measures, and also choose the most appropriate procedure.

WANEBO and QUAN (1974) reported 18 failures of electrocoagulation for primary carcinoma of the rectum, referred to the Memorial Hospital after treatment elsewhere. Only nine patients could undergo a curative excision; the other nine had advanced lesions suitable for palliative treatment alone, and died from cancer. Of the 14 patients followed up over 5 years, only three survived disease-free (21%). The authors conclude that the poor results after electrocoagulation were related to two main causes: (a) the wrong indications for conservative treatment, which was performed for deeply invasive rectal cancer, or cancer with regional lymph node metastasis; (b) the long interval between the first electrocoagulation and the tentative salvage treatment.

This experience emphasizes the responsibility of the clinician – surgeon or radiotherapist – who initiates conservative treatment for a patient with a clinically limited rectal cancer. He must bear in mind that such lesions can usually be cured by major surgery.

3. Follow-up

Careful follow-up must always be maintained after conservative treatment, in constrast to that after AP excision for rectal cancer, since local recurrence within the pelvis or perineum is rarely suitable to further curative surgery. Such patients are only suitable for palliative measures, and the patients will eventually die from cancer whatever treatment is applied and even if the recurrence has been detected early.

After local treatment, patients must be followed up regularly and carefully in order to detect local or regional failures as early as possible. Many recurrences can be treated effectively by major surgery, and a number of patients will be cured. Experience from this type of follow-up has shown that there are two types of failure: some represent extensions of highly malignant disease and are usually accompanied by peritoneal, lymphatic, or liver dissemination. Other grow slowly and remain localized for a period which may allow a salvage operation if they are detected early.

Follow-up consists of digital and endoscopic examination, which may be combined with cytological examination of scrape smears from the treated area. It should be done by the original surgeon or radiotherapist because he will remember all the details of the case history and of the tumour configuration and location, and he will be in a better position to observe early changes in the treated area and to decide on the need for surgery. The CEA test is not of great help after local treatment of limited rectal cancer, because it is usually negative. However, it is advisable to do this test twice a year during the first 3 years after conservative treatment. Unfortunately, a positive CEA test indicates extensive and incurable recurrence in most cases. Clinical follow-up examination should take place at least every 2 months during the first year, every 3 months during the second year every 6 months during the next 3 years, and once a year after the 5th year. Most failures occur during the first 2 years, but late recurrences are not exceptional and the clinician should be in touch with the patient for a long period of time.

4. Modalities of Conservative Treatment for Rectal Cancer

Most statistics for rectal cancer treated by surgery contain about 15% of DUKES' A cases at the time of diagnosis, and these cases are theorectically suitable for conservative treatment. Several techniques may be used for conservative treatment of rectal cancers, either surgical or radiotherapeutic. In all cases, the purpose of the conservative treatment is to cure the patient by controlling the primary tumour separately from its lymphatic drainage and without resection of bowel. To embark upon a conservative course with a cure in mind, the operator – surgeon or radiotherapist – must follow rigid guidelines in patient selection and in application of the treatment procedure. Otherwise this aim will not be achieved and the best management will not be provided. Conservative treatment can be carried out by surgery or by radiation therapy.

Every technique has its own effectiveness, its own advantages and complications. It is justifiable to analyse the possibilities of each method and compare them with regard to the chances of cure and the disadvantages involved. Special attention should be paid to the morbidity due to treatment, since a high percentage of the patients treated conservatively are those in poor general condition.

V. Conservative Treatment by Surgery

There are three modalities of local surgery: local excision, electrocoagulation, and cryosurgery.

1. Local Excision

Local excision is now regarded as a possible alternative to radical resection in carefully selected patients. MORSON et al. (1977) conceives this operation as a "total biopsy", which is followed by a thorough histological examination of the specimen to ascertain whether removal of the cancer was complete and whether the presence of other histological criteria might indicate further radical surgery.

Local excision usually comprises the removal of a full-thickness segment of the rectal wall underlying the tumour, together with an adequate surrounding cuff of normal tissue. The method most commonly used is a per- or transanal approach using a suitable anal retractor or a wide-bore sigmoidoscope. Sometimes the tumour can be prolapsed through the anal canal by traction. This technique is referred to as the "parachute" method in France, when wires passed through the rectal wall adjacent to tumour are used to deliver it.

The transsphincteric approach has been popularized by MASON (1974, 1980). This author has pointed out that the "sphincter can be divided completely to provide an excellent exposure of the interior of the rectum and, contrary to long-accepted tradition, if sutured accurately it heals well and patients regain normal defecation with full anal continence". When an early cancer has been defined by pre-operative clinical staging, MASON obtains a direct view of anterior tumours by division of the sphincter after a posterior approach, and then carries out an elliptical excision using surgical diathermy. The defect is closed transversely with a single layer of interrupted suture. For growths situated higher-up in the rectum, the technique is the same, and the rectovesical or rectovaginal pouch is entered without difficulty. MASON (1974, 1980) modified his technique for posterior quadrant growths; the division of the anal canal and rectum is stopped short of the lower edge of the tumour. The posterior wall is then mobilized through the pararectal space, so that the growth can be prolapsed into the lumen and seen face on.

For more invasive cancers, which are still confined to the rectal wall, MASON advises resection of a closed tube of rectum with restoration of continuity by end-to-end anastomis. KRASKE's posterior approach and the transvaginal approach are less commonly used. Patients treated by simple transanal excision do not need a temporary colostomy, but a temporary defunctioning colostomy, established at the time of the local excision, is advisable for most patients treated by the posterior approach.

There appears to be little difference in the outcome for the patients treated by different types of local surgery, and the choice of approach depends on the preference and experience of the surgeon and on the location of the tumour. All these approaches are characterized by removal of the tumour with a small margin of normal bowel for safety, and without removal of regional lymph nodes.

Careful pathological study of the specimen and close collaboration between surgeon and pathologist are required in all cases. LOCK et al. have pointed out that any surgeon undertaking local excision for rectal cancer must not only select the tumours carefully, but also have the help of an experienced pathologist. Careful histological examination of the operative specimen includes an assessment of several features: (a) depth of invasion of the rectal wall by carcinoma, (b) completeness of local excision, and (c) grade of malignancy of the invasive carcinoma.

The interpretation of the pathological report by the surgeon must leave him with no doubt that the tumour has been completely excised, and until such a time the specimen should be regarded as an excision biopsy. Personal discussion between clinician and pathologist should be sought whereever possible, and this is mandatory if either believes that excision has been incomplete. LOCK et al. (1978) add that "tumors excised by diathermy present a particular problem, because a narrow zone of tissue at the line of section is destroyed. Thus the surgeon may believe the tumor to be excised incompletely, while the pathologist reports excision has been complete".

If there is a doubt about the total excision of the lesion, or if the tumour proves to be colloid or poorly differentiated, then further radical surgery should be performed without delay.

The experience at St. Marks's Hospital in the field of local excision deserves special attention. Between 1948 and 1972, the percentage of local excisions gradually increased from under 1% to over 9%. During this period 110 cancers of the rectum were treated by this procedure, but the figure gives a false impression because most of these tumours (88) were pedunculated adenomas with focal areas of malignancy. The real problem concerns the non-pedunculated sessile adenocarcinomas. Between 1948 and 1978, 42 cases were treated at St. Mark's Hospital, and reported by LOCK et al. (1978) and by HAWLEY and RITCHIE (1980). There were 22 protuberant tumours, and 20 ulcerated tumours. The results are reported in Table 3.

Subsequent histological examination showed that 14% of cases were not suitable for local excision, and late recurrence was observed in 20%. In 1964, CARDEN and MORSON from the same institution reported a series of 40 patients with pedunculated or non-pedunculated malignant polyps of the rectum, with a 17.5% incidence of late recurrence. Of these seven cases with recurrent-tumours four patients died from cancer and one died after further surgery.

In 1973, WILSON from Sydney reported a series of 30 patients treated by local excision, with only two recurrences in both of which further local treatment was

Table 3. Results of local excision for rectal cancer (HAWLEY (1981)

No. of cases	42 (follow-up from 1 to 30 years)
Early reoperation	6 (14%) (4 colostomies)
No early further treatment after local excision	36
Late recurrence	7 (20%) (3 colostomies)
Nodes involved	3
Post-operative death	1
Death from cancer	2 (5.5%)

Table 4. Local excision for rectal carcinoma (HERMANEK 1980)

	Local excision considered as sufficient procedure	Radical surgery indicated but not performed
No. of cases	48	23
Mean follow-up time (months)	33	37
Local recurrence	5 (10%)	10 (43%)
Distant metastasis	2 (4%)	5 (22%)
Cancer death	1 (2%)	4 (17%)

successful. MASON (1976b) mentioned two local recurrences in a series of 41 cases. HERMANEK et al. (1980; Erlangen, Germany) has recently published a carefully selected series of 71 rectal cancers treated by local excision. The patients were divided into two groups: 48 cases for which local excision was considered a sufficient procedure, and 23 cases for which radical surgery was indicated on the basis of pathological examination, but not performed because of poor general condition, advanced age, or refusal by the patient. In the selected group, the rate of local recurrence was 10% versus 43% in the unfavourable group. The rate of cancer death was 4% versus 17%. These results are analysed in Table 4.

There are two types of local recurrence: some recurrences are due to incomplete removal of neoplastic tissue, and are cured by a wider excision. Others are related to highly malignant and diffuse disease and are unlikely to be cured even if radical surgery is undertaken. It should also be remembered that local recurrence may occur following excision of pedunculated adenocarcinomas with invasion of the stalk.

Selection of the cases to be treated by local excision alone is made on two grounds. After clinical selection a further 14% of the cases treated at the St. Mark's Hospital are excluded on histological criteria. In spite of this double selection, the rate of local recurrence is between 10% and 15%. In Chapter V the use of elective irradiation to decrease the incidence of local recurrence after local excision will be discussed.

If one takes into consideration the criteria of selection, local excision appears less simple than it might seem at first glance, and in all cases it requires a close collaboration between surgeon and experienced pathologist. If this collaboration does not exist – if the surgeon is not exactly aware of the details of the pathologist's interpretation – local excision becomes hazardous and can fail to control the tumour. However, with proper selection local excision can be a curative procedure which merits a place in the treatment of polypoid rectal cancers.

2. Electrocoagulation

Until 20 years ago electrocoagulation was with few exceptions reserved for palliation in the treatment of inoperable rectal cancers, but it has now become an accepted treatment for cure of selected cancers of the rectum. STRAUSS et al. (1935, Chicago) in 1913 were the first to apply electrocoagulation to tumours of the rectum, initially for palliation and later for cure. Electrocoagulation implies deep destruction of the tumour and adjacent tissue by heat. Electrocoagulation must be distinguished from fulguration, which is defined as destruction of tissue by sparking and implies destruction of superficial lesions only. Many reports have been published and the most important include the series of JACKMAN (1961), POIRIER (1969), CRILE and TURNBULL (1972), SWERDLOW and SALVATI (1972), KRATZER and ONSANIT (1972), SALVATI and RUBIN (1976), and MADDEN (1979).

Techniques, indications, and selection of the cases suitable for electrocoagulation vary somewhat according to the operators, and it is difficult to compare results. The procedure is usually conducted with the patient in the lithotomy position (or in the prone position advised by MADDEN and KANDALAFT (1967; 1971 a, b) for tumours of the anterior wall). Caudal anaesthesia is performed to obtain adequate relaxation of the sphincter. The exposure of the tumour is the key to electrocoagulation. If good exposure cannot be obtained, electrocoagulation is contra-indicated and must not be attempted. A bivalved anal speculum is used by CULP (1976) to allow exposure of the lesion. A large operating proctoscope, equipped with suction to remove the smoke, is used by CRILE and TURNBULL (1972). MADDEN and KANDALAFT dilate the anus by the progressive introduction of from two to five fingers. Then a Harrington retractor is used to obtain good exposure of the whole lesion. MADDEN and KANDALAFT (1967; 1971 a, b) use a needlepoint electrode inserted into the tissue, whereas CRILE and TURNBULL 1972 "use a brass wire loop about 1 cm in diameter. The cancerous tissue is destroyed by heat, it crumbles and is wiped away whereas muscle chars to the consistency of leather. Fat is easily recognized by color and by the sizzling that is produced when it is heated". MADDEN (1979) repeats electrocoagulation and scraping of the coagulated tissue until a soft pliable base is noted on palpation. A final fulguration is then done. A dry gauze sponge is inserted, the end of which protrudes through the anus. The sponge is removed after 3 h.

As a supplementary method, irradiation was used by several authors: JACKMAN (1961) used radium therapy in 20% of cases; CRILE and TURNBULL (1972) implantation of radon seeds or cobalt therapy in 20% of cases; CULP (1976), radium plates in 50% of cases. This application of irradiation was carried out during the original treatment, or delayed until the coagulation slough had begun to separate.

After the initial treatment, the patient may remain in hospital for 1 week (JACKMAN 1961, SWERDLOW and SALVATI 1972). MADDEN's patients remain at least 2 weeks in hospital and they are anaesthesized a second time while the operative area is inspected and palpated. Biopsies of representative areas are obtained and electrocoagulation is again performed. Seven to 10 days later the patient is discharged and instructed to return at monthly intervals. It is also emphasized that during the ensuing 6 months, admission to the hospital is dependent upon the findings of follow-up examinations. Generally two readmissions will be necessary. Early detection of residual deposits and their immediate treatment are essential for the success of the method. The number of electrocoagulations varies from one to 13, the average being four sessions for each patient. Of MADDEN's patients 13.7% had only one session, 60% had two or three sessions, 18.9% five to seven sessions, and 7.4% between eight and 13 sessions.

The rate of complications reported varies greatly with different authors. JACKMAN (1961) does not mention iatrogenic morbidity. CRILE and TURNBULL (1972), and SWERDLOW and SALVATI (1972) note that delayed bleeding occurred occasionally after the eschar had separated, but that it always responded to conservative management, stopped spontaneously, and never needed recoagulation of a vessel.

In contrast, 24.5% of the patients treated by MADDEN (1979) developed complications related to the electrocoagulation: haemorrhage occured in 29 patients (16.6% of cases), requiring subsequent haemostatic coagulation in 16 cases; there were also four rectovaginal fistulas and two perforations into the peritoneal cavity.

If the coagulated area is large, a stricture may develop. These strictures are managed by periodic dilatations in the surgery (SWERDLOW and SALVATI 1972). CRILE and TURNBULL (1972) did not see a stricture which required a permanent colostomy and MADDEN (1979) reported four strictures.

a) Results

The Mayo Clinic Experience. The results of electrocoagulation for early rectal cancers at the Mayo Clinic have been reported in a series of publications. In 1958, WITTOESCH and JACKMAN (1958) reported their experience with 128 cases (1945–1949) which were treated by conservative procedures instead of major surgery according to several protocols: fulguration, irradiation by radium, a combination of the two, or local excision. Out of the 116 patients followed over 5 years, 54 (46%) had lived 5 years or more after treatment. Of the 75 patients who did not survive 5 years 30 died of cancer, and 24 of the deaths were known to be unrelated to cancer.

In 1961, JACKMAN reported a group of 252 patients seen from 1941 till 1952 and considered to be suitable for conservative treatment: 211 were treated by electrocoagulation, 50.8% being grade I adenocarcinoma in an adenoma, 34.5% grade I adenocarcinoma, 13.1% grade II adenocarcinoma, and 1.3% grade III adenocarcinoma. The other 41 cases were treated by radical surgery. All tumours were sessile and had dimensions of 2 cm or more in their greatest diameter. More than half on the lesions were on the posterior rectal wall, and almost all tumours were below the peritoneal reflexion. Deaths and complications from intercurrent disease occurred, but as far as could be ascertained 96.2% of 211 patients were cured.

Conservative treatment was considered to have failed in eight patients (3.8%). Three of these eight patients were found to have induration or tumours beneath the scar of the fulgurated site. These local recurrences were detected at intervals of 6 months to 2½ years after the initial conservative treatment. A combined AP resection was then carried out. Three patients have survived for 8, 10, and 11 years apparently free from cancer, and are considered partial failures only.

The other five patients died from cancer. Four of the five underwent a combined AP operation, which demonstrated the presence of extensive metastasis. One refused surgery. In three cases, the original pathology had revealed grade 1 adenocarcinoma in an adenoma. In the other two, the lesions were grade 1 adenocarcinoma.

In 1974, CULP and JACKMAN reviewed a series of 80 patients treated by conservative measures. Fifty-nine tumours were considered operable, 21 were rejected as unsuitable. There were 18 (30%) treatment failures; 12 patients in the group died of cancer, three were alive and well following radical surgery for the recurrent disease, and three died of unrelated causes. In this series, 38 of 80 patients (48%) were alive and well 5 years after conservative treatment.

In 1976, CULP published a series of 67 patients with rectal adenocarcinomas located in the distal 6 cm of the rectum, of which 48 were operable, 19 were considered inoperable, 28 tumours were polypoid, and 39 were ulcerative. Sixty-one were grade 1 or 11, four were grade 111, and two were grade IV. In 37 cases radium plaques were applied to the treated area as a supplementary method either immediately or a few days after conservative surgery. Of the 67 patients, 46 were alive at 5 years (overall survival rate of 69%); 17 of the remaining 21 were treatment failures (25%), the other four having died of intercurrent disease. Of these 17 patients, 11 died of rectal cancer, one patient died post-operatively, two were cured by subsequent radical surgery, and three died of unrelated causes.

The Cleveland Clinic Experience. In 1972, CRILE and TURNBULL reported a selected group of 62 cases treated by electrocoagulation with a 5-year survival rate of 69%. They compared this group to another group of 220 patients treated by AP resection at the same period by the same surgeons, with a 5-year cure rate of 46%. Several comments must be made about this comparison of the results of two methods of treatment:
1. All tumours located high enough to be treated by anterior resection or pull-through procedures, as well as lesions that involved the anus, were excluded.
2. The average diameter of the tumours treated by resection was 1.7 cm greater than those treated by coagulation (4.8 cm versus 3.1 cm).
3. The configuration of the tumours treated by coagulation was associated with a more favourable prognosis than those treated by resection (44% versus 26% polypoid-type tumours, 56% versus 71% ulcerating tumours).
4. The average age was greater in the group of patients whose tumours were treated locally (67 years) than those treated radically (61 years).

5. The immediate and delayed operative mortality rate of resection was 5%, whereas there was no mortality related to the coagulation.

To compensate for the difference in size of the tumours in the two groups the patients were compared in randomized matched pairs. This was accomplished by matching each patient treated by coagulation with another patient who had a tumour of the same size treated by radical excision. The comparison of 46 matched pairs shows that the 5-year survival rate was 67% (31/46) in the coagulation group, versus 54% (25/46) in the resection group.

CRILE and TURNBULL (1972) recognized that it was difficult to compare the configurations of the tumours in the two groups. In those patients treated by coagulation, the classification was established by proctoscopic examination only, whereas in the other group the configuration could be appreciated more easily in the operative specimen. These authors considered that the rectum could still be removed with prospects of cure as good as if it had been resected initially in the 13% of patients in whom the carcinoma was not controlled locally. In the discussion, they dealt with the major problem of lymphatic spread, which remains the main argument in favour of radical surgery. They noted that only a third of the patients treated by resection had metastases in nodes, and that only a fifth of the patients who had nodal metastases were permanently cured, so that 15 patients had to undergo operation before one patient with curable metastases in lymph nodes was included. In their opinion, resection by removing nodes increased the rate of cure of the entire group by only 7%. They considered that local treatment by electrocoagulation was a satisfactory alternative to radical surgery for carcinoma of the lower rectum up to 5 cm in diameter, especially in poor surgical risk patient. The 5-year survival rate was 93% (25/27) for polypoid tumours, and 51% (18/35) for ulcerating tumours.

Experience at St. Clare's Hospital, New York City. (MADDEN 1979, MADDEN and KANDALAFT 1961, 1971 b) From 1954 up to February 1977, MADDEN and KANDALAFT (1967) treated 175 patients with rectal cancer by electrocoagulation. The average age of the patient was 68.6 years, and 41.1% of the patients were 70 or older. Most rectal cancers (70.3%) were located in the lower third of the rectum between 2 cm and 6 cm from the anal verge, 22.8% were located between 7 cm and 10 cm, and 6.3% (three squamous cell carcinomas, eight adenocarcinomas) were situated in the anal area. Of these tumours 74,3% were limited because their size did not exceed 4 cm, 18.3% were larger than 5 cm (up to 7 cm), and 5.7% were annular. The number of sessions of electrocoagulation depended on the size of the tumour. The average duration of each session of electrocoagulation was 1 h 20 min. Of the 175 tumours treated by electrocoagulation, 30 were not true rectal cancers but villous tumours with malignant change, 63 were polypoid adenocarcinomas, 63 were ulcerative carcinomas, and ten were stenosing lesions. One hundred and twenty-eight patients (73.1%) were considered operable, 47 (26.9%) inoperable.

The long-term results were as follows:
Cure: 93 (53.1%); follow-up from 2 to 22 years
Deaths from cancer: 47 (26.9%); follow-up from 0.5 to 9 years
Deaths from other causes (five with cancer): 29 (16.6%); follow-up from 0.2 to 13 years

Table 5. Relation between type of tumour and survival rate (MADDEN 1979)

	No. of cases	Cured	Cure rate
Villous tumour	30	19	63.3%
Polypoid tumour	63	40	63.5%
Ulcerated tumour	63	31	55.2%
Stenosing tumour	10	1	6.2%
	166	91	54.8%

Lost to follow-up: 6 (3.4%).

One hundred and three patients were followed up for over 5 years: Of the 73 originally considered operable, 51 were cured (5-year survival rate, i.e. no evidence of disease = 69.9%); of the 30 originally considered inoperable, 11 were cured (5-year survival rate = 36.7%). The cure rate was related to the configuration of the lesion, as Table 5 shows.

Experience of Poirier (1969; Angouleme, France). Of 80 rectal adenocarcinomas treated with a follow-up greater than 5 years, 44 (55%) were cured, 25 (31%) were considered failures, and 11 patients were lost to follow-up. Another group of 31 patients with malignant change in villous tumours were treated by electrocoagulation, with success in 41%.

Experience of Van Slooten and Van Dobbenburgh (1980, Amsterdam). VAN SLOOTEN and VAN DOBBENBURGH have emphasized the advantages of fulguration. Short sparks heat the tissue to such a degree that evaporation of all the elements occurs without any charring. With this technique it is possible to recognize all the structures in the treated area: mucosa, submucosa, circular and longitudinal muscle, perirectal fat, tumour strands, and blood-vessels, and the depth of infiltration can be quite accurately defined.

A series of 60 cases is divided into two groups: 43 cases in which the rules of selection were followed, and 17 cases in which there was a transgression of these rules. The overall 5-year survival NED (no evidence of disease) rate was 66% (40 of 60 cases). In the group of 43 cases, eight (18%) local recurrences occurred and presacral nodes were involved in six cases; 31 (72%) patients were alive and well at 5 years. In the group of 17 cases, five local recurrences occurred; nine (52%) patients were alive and well at 5 years, two of them after radical surgery.

To summarize, one must stress that the results published in these series differ markedly when one considers the cures, the failures and the proportion salvaged by surgery after the failure of electrocoagulation (Table 6).

Many of these differences can be explained by the selection of the cases suitable for coagulation. First of all, malignant change in villous tumours and grade 1 adenocarcinomas in adenomas, which represented 50.8% of tumours in the series of JACKMAN (1961) and 18% in the series of MADDEN, (1979) should not be compared with true invasive rectal adenocarcinomas. The number of ulcerative tumours, which require destruction of a substantial thickness of the rectal wall, will reduce the chance of local control and increase the risk of complications such as haemorrhage and stricture.

Table 6. Statistics for electrocoagulation

Author	No. of cases	Cure rate	Rate of local failure	Proportion of control by subsequent surgery
CULP and JACKMAN (1974)	80	48%	30%	6/18
CULP (1976)	67	69%	25%	6/17
MADDEN (1979)	175	53.1%	23%	3/9
CRILE and TURNBULL (1972)	62	68%	13%	7/8
POIRIER (1969)	80	55%	31%	
KRATZER and ONSANIT (1972)	27	15%		0/2
WILSON (1973)	30		7%	2/2
SALVATI and RUBIN (1976)	51		47%	7/17
WANEBO and QUAN (1974)				3/14

The ability of electrocoagulation to control limited rectal cancers, especially the protuberant and ulcerative slightly infiltrating tumours, has been demonstrated.

A final point which must be mentioned is the observation by STRAUSS (1969) that destruction by surgical diathermy of the major portion of a cancer of the rectum is sometimes followed by spontaneous regression of the remainder of the cancer. It is claimed that the products of tissue necrosis are absorbed slowly and act as antigens which stimulate host resistance. This theory that electrocoagulation evokes an immune reponse has no experimental basis. MADDEN (1979) quoted the work of MORTON at the National Institute of Health (NIH), who studied blood serum samples from patients before and after treatment of the rectal tumour by electrocoagulation. However, he was unable to detect any specific antibody reaction or auto-immune reponse in these patients. The only finding was that of a non-specific antibody reaction, and so far it has not been demonstrated that effectiveness of electrocoagulation can be ascribed to an immunological basis.

3. Cryosurgery

Cryosurgery is the destruction of tissue by the application of very low temperature probes. It has been used as a means of treating certain anorectal diseases. The operation is performed with a cryoprobe tip fixed to a hand-held instrument, attached by tubing to a cylinder of nitrous oxide or liquid nitrogen. The cryoprobe tip is designed to operate in direct contact with the tissues to be destroyed. The procedure may be performed in the surgery or, more usually, in a hospital operating-room. It requires local anesthesia and good exposure of the lesion.

The method has been used mainly in the treatment of haemorrhoids as an alternative to local excision. There are very few publications about the application of cryosurgery to rectal adenocarcinoma. LANGER and BROCKAMP (1980) reported a series of 162 cases of rectal cancer treated by cryosurgery since 1972: 58 patients were inoperable because of their general condition (group A); 65 were inoperable because of the local extent of the disease, distant metastasis, or recurrence after anterior resection (group B); 12 refused to undergo an AP resection; and 27 underwent cryotherapy as a pre-operative procedure. In 16 cases complications occurred: six episodes of haemorrhage, three perforations, and seven stenoses. Of the 47 determinate group A patients (i.e. those who were followed up and did not die from other causes), 14 survived more than 2 years and 10 more than 3 years. Of the 51 determinate group B patients, 21 survived more than 2 years and 11 more than 3 years. LANGER and BROCKAMP (1980) admits that there is very little evidence to suggest that cryotherapy has more than a non-specific influence on the host's immunity, similar to that which follows electrocoagulation.

KNOCK and KOBERNICK (1978) reported on the results of cryosurgery in 18 patients: eight had rectal adenocarcinomas, ten had malignant change in villous tumours. All patients were poor-risk or inoperable. In those with rectal cancer, the results were poor and only palliative; control of the lesion was rarely obtained. In the patients with villous tumours, cryosurgery was applied to the bed of the lesion after local excision as a supplementary method to improve the chance of local control.

OSBORNE et al. (1978), and FEIFEL and LETZER (1980) consider that cryosurgery does not appear to be acceptable as an alternative to excision or resection, even in the early stages of rectal carcinoma, and that the indication for cryotherapy should be restricted to pàlliative treatment. At the moment there are technical problems which limit the application of cryosurgery to rectal tumours in certain situations. It is too early to see if it will have a well-defined role because its use has not yet demonstrated any improvement over established surgical or radiotherapeutic techniques.

VI. Conservative Treatment by Irradiation

It may seem surprising that during the past 10 years radiation therapy has acquired a significant place in the local treatment for cure of carcinoma of the rectum. Rectal cancer is generally considered to be only slightly radiosensitive, and it is admitted that radiation therapy per se is unable to control rectal tumours. This judgement is based on the poor efficacy of irradiation when applied to advanced tumours or to recurrences after surgery.

The rectum is at the same time a deep and an accessible organ. It is deeply situated in the pelvis, far from the skin surface, protected by pelvic bones, and close to structures which are very sensitive to irradiation. It is, however, possible to gain direct access to the rectum through the anus. Accordingly, irradiation may be applied to rectal cancer by two routes: (a) external irradiation, which is essentially used in pre- and post-operative or palliative situations: and (b) intracavitary irradiation, the only reliable procedure for the cure of rectal cancer.

1. Historical Background

For several decades, roentgentherapy was limited to levels under 250 kV (conventional or orthovoltage roentgentherapy). The mean distance between the skin and the rectum is at least 10 cm, so that the dose distributed to the rectum in conventional roentgentherapy was less than one-fourth of the skin dose. The radiotherapist was forced to get an adequate dose to the deep tissues by the artifice of cross-fire. In spite of these therapeutic modalities, 200-kV roentgentherapy had almost no effect on carcinoma of the rectum, which was considered radioresistant.

By 1929, REGAUD (1929) had already observed that there were three difficulties in the irradiation of rectal tumours. The first was that the tumour cells were scarcely more radiosensitive than those of the surrounding normal rectal mucosa; the second was that the growth was often so extensive that uniform irradiation was difficult or impossible to achieve; and the third was that good access to the growth was hard to obtain. In the absence of success with conventional roentgentherapy many authors tried to treat rectal tumours by a direct approach per anum with radium.

In 1914, SYMONDS reported the first case of rectal adenocarcinoma treated with radium. At the time of surgical excision, 7 months later, no residual tumour was found. Since that time, there have been many publications concerning intracavitary or/and interstitial radium therapy: most results were palliative. Some patients developed severe complications, but a few good results from these methods and clinical cures lasting over 5 years have been described by FINZI (1950), FITZWILLIAMS (1939, eight cases), CADE (1950, three cases), BERTILLON and WERNER (1933), and RENAUX (1933).

MAISIN and LANGEROCK (1953) used long needles (4 or 5 cm), inserted with special forceps through a proctoscope. The needles were implanted at 45 ° to the long axis of the rectum, after a ring had been placed in the uppermost part of the growth, and then as the proctoscope was withdrawn second and third rings were inserted as required. The needles were left in place for 48–72 h. MAISIN and LANGEROCK also combined the intracavitary treatment with external X-ray therapy, and reported 25 patients who survived 5 years. A colostomy was necessary in all cases.

At the Christie Hospital, Manchester, another method reported by PATERSON (1963) consisted of implanting long needles through the peri-anal skin. The needles were enclosed in long sheaths of monel metal, so that the total active length was as great as 10 cm. Six to eight of these containers were arranged cylindrically around the rectum, and a cavitary applicator was inserted into its lumen. The combination, if accurately placed, gave a field of reasonably homogeneous radiation of which the intensity could be calculated. The needles were left in place for 5–7 days, but the dose was so arranged that the cavitary tube could be removed after 3–4 days,. A total dose of 6000 rad could be achieved. The treatment was a major undertaking associated with a definite mortality; it was repeated once or even twice for some patients. Ten per cent of 5-year cures were reported, and these were for the most part early cases in which operation was contra-indicated for various reasons.

BINKLEY (1928, 1938) at the Memorial Hospital described the selective use of irradiation in the treatment of rectal cancer for cure in poor-risk patients. The sources of radiation included insertions of radium or radon seeds and external irradiation in a series of 18 patients with small tumours. Eighty-three per cent were locally controlled.

In 1961, RUFF et al. from the Mayo Clinic reported a series of 96 rectal cancers treated between 1914 and 1943 with radium and subsequent excision 6 weeks or more after completion of irradiation. The technique of irradiation and the doses distributed varied widely. Radium was used in interstitial insertion in 13 cases, or in surface application in 83 cases. In ten cases, no residual carcinoma was found in the operative specimen. The authors concluded that radium could sometimes completely destroy an adenocarcinoma of the rectum.

During the past 3 decades, significant progress has been made in the field of radiation therapy with the development of supervoltage irradiation (cobalt-60, X-rays of high energy), new machines for delivery of intracavitary roentgentherapy, replacement of radium by iridium-192 in interstitial curietherapy, and computerized dosimetry.

2. External Beam Irradiation

False hopes were raised by supervoltage irradiation with the greater penetration of the X-ray or gammy-ray beams, and the phenomenon of build-up. High doses of radiation can be delivered to a deeply seated tumour such as rectal cancer, without skin reaction and with better protection of the surrounding structures. However, the advent of high-energy radiations has deceived those who expected that their use would make tumours more radiosensitive. Modern external irradiation applied to large, unresectable rectal tumours or to recurrences after surgery has contributed to palliation but not to cure in most cases. Pain has been relieved and there has been a decrease in bleeding and mucous discharge, but not a significant increase in patient survival.

WILLIAMS and HORWITZ (1956) reported in 1956 a series of 189 patients treated at St. Bartholomew's Hospital, London, from 1937–1954, with roentgen rays generated at 1000 kV as external irradiation. The dose delivered was 6000 rad to the whole of the tumour-bearing volume over 6–8 weeks. The crude 5-year survival rate was 4.7%. Of nine patients alive at 5 years, two were in the group of 26 with tumours thought to be confined to the rectal wall, and seven were in the group of 115 with lesions which had spread beyond the rectum to neighbouring structures and/or involved regional lymph nodes. Of these nine patients three survived more than 10 years, four died from intercurrent disease, and two patients died of their cancer. More recently, WANG and SCHULZ (1962) reported seven patients who survived for 4–15 years, without disease, following the administration of 3500–5500 rad to their tumour.

The reports of experience with pre-operative irradiation illustrate the poor control of the disease by modern external irradiation alone. In the series reported by STEVENS et al. (1976) 97 patients were treated pre-operatively with a dose of 5000 rad of cobalt-60 over 5 weeks. The patient underwent major surgery more than 1 month later. In ten cases (10.3%) there was no residual tumour in the operative specimen and the adenocarcinoma was entirely destroyed by irradiation.

Critical examination of the results reported by various workers using external irradiation suggests that, in the majority of patients treated, tumour destruction by external irradiation alone occurred only with tumours which were superficial and confined to the bowel wall, or when the tumour was espacially radiosensitive. It must be added that it is impossible to predict the response to external irradiation in any one individual case. In 1963, PATERSON in his book *Treatment of Malignant Diseases by Radiotherapy* gave his opinion on external radiotherapy and expressed a pessimistic point of view with the exception of limited rectal tumours, which can be treated directly by intracavitary or interstitial procedures.

At the present time, with the types of radiation commonly used in teletherapy (gamma rays of cobalt-60, high energy X-rays of linear accelerator), it is admitted that external irradiation is not a reliable procedure to control rectal adenocarcinoma, whereas intrarectal methods of irradiation have proved to be much more efficient in selected cases.

3. Intracavitary Irradiation of Rectal Tumours

The term "intracavitary irradiation" in its limited sense is applied to irradiation given by means of an X-ray or gamma-ray emitter located in the lumen of the rectum. Practically it seems better no include under this heading not only true intracavitary irradiation, but also interstitial curietherapy, which is performed by the transanal route with direct insertion into the rectal wall. The latter may be regarded as a supplementary technique.

If one accepts this definition, there are two modalities of intracavitary irradiation: contact X-ray therapy and interstitial curietherapy.

a) Contact X-ray Therapy

The principles of contact X-ray therapy were laid down by CHAOUL (1936, Berlin). Two conditions are required: (a) short focal distance, i.e. distance between the X-ray focus and the object; and (b) soft radiation quality.

In 1932, SCHAEFER and WITTE devised a tube with an anode at one end for insertion into a cavity such as the vagina, to treat carcinoma of the uterine cervix. Owing to the shortage of radium in Germany, CHAOUL (1936) developed the use of a short focal-target distance on the grounds that the distribution of the energy absorbed in the tissues was the important factor in the radium treatment, and not the quality of the radiation. CHAOUL, who was really the pioneer in the development of this technique, aimed at producing conditions for the use of X-rays which would approximate, in certain respects, to those of radium therapy. CHAOUL and WACHSMANN (1953) called this method *Nahbestrahlung,* i.e. short focal distance irradiation, most commonly known as contact X-ray therapy. This name, though not strictly accurate, does, as pointed out by BROMLEY (1938), serve to emphasize the limitation of this form of treatment. Short-distance X-ray therapy is essentially a method of treating accessible lesions that can be brought directly into contact with the applicator of the tube without interposition of normal tissues.

In contact X-ray therapy, a very steep dose drop is of great importance; otherwise it would not be possible to administer a high radiation dose to superficial pathological tissue without also irradiating healthy normal tissue located beneath it.

Use of the Siemens Machine. The first short focal distance, low-voltage X-ray therapy machine was built by SIEMENS. This unit works at 60 kV constant potential and 4 mA. The total filtration is equivalent to 0.2 mm nickel and commonly employed focal target distances are 5 cm and 7 cm. Isodose curves for a 4-cm diameter circular field at a focal distance of 5 cm show that 50% of the energy is delivered at a depth of 17 mm, and that at 3 cm depth there remains only 28% of the surface dose.

Besides the treatment of skin tumours, this method was originally planned by CHAOUL in 1934 for the application of X-rays to tumours of the rectum, which had been exposed by a posterior surgical approach as follows: (a) colostomy; (b) surgical access to the posterior wall of the rectum with successive resection of the coccyx and the lowest part of the sacrum, mobilization of the rectum, and incision of the rectal wall and suture of it to the skin; (c) direct sequential irradiation on the exposed tumour; (d) closure of the sacral access; and (e) closure of the colostomy.

A few years later, CHAOUL (1936) was prompted by some encouraging results to discard operative exposure of the growth and to start intracavitary transanal X-ray therapy for rectal cancers. The introduction of a special speculum with a light allowed him to select the fields for treatment. Once the rectoscope was positioned with the patient in the knee-chest position, the X-ray applicator was passed through the rectoscope. The X-ray tube was relatively heavy and not portable. It was locked to an arm bound to the generator. During the application of radiotherapy, the operator was separated from the patient by a lead glass screen. The treatment consisted of three series of ten to 12 daily applications on two to four fields. The daily dose was 400–500 R, the total dose 14000–16000 R over a period of 56–88 days. Each course of irradiation was separated from the following one by an interval of 10 days.

The X-ray tube commonly used by CHAOU had an anode of the transmission target type, adapted to tumours of limited extent and suitable contour. CHAOUL invented another tube with a conical terminal anode, suitable for annular growths. With this SIEMENS unit, CHAOUL and WACHSMANN (1953) claimed to have treated more than 100 rectal cancers, many of them unresectable. In 62 cases primary healing followed the irradiation, and there was a satisfactory response after 4 years in a considerable number, but no details of the cases were described.

In their book *Die Nahbestrahlung,* CHAOUL and WACHSMANN (1953) reported on 30 patients cured with a follow-up of 4–17 years. In the analysis of these results, however, it must be kept in mind that many patients treated by CHAOUL and WACHSMANN had advanced lesions, or were considered inoperable.

LARRÙ (1957, Madrid) reported on a series of 46 patients treated with the CHAOUL technique: 11 operable, 28 inoperable, and seven advanced cases. He noted 25 patients (54%) cured for 2–7 years. Fifteen patients died from cancer, four from intercurrent disease, and two post-operatively.

However, the SIEMENS machine was not well adapted to intrarectal applications, and the CHAOUL technique of irradiation of rectal tumours was abandoned in the 1950s.

Use of the Philips Machine. A second great departure in contact X-ray therapy was made by VAN DER PLAATS (1938), who designed the PHILIPS machine (Eindhoven, Holland). This unit, called RT 50, built for the treatment of skin cancers, is particularly well adapted to intracavitary applications (Fig. 10).

By contrast with the SIEMENS tube, which is a transmission target type, the X-rays passing through the material of the anode to reach the tumour, the design of the PHILIPS tube is essentially that of an early diagnosis tube, with a ring filament and solid anode. The X-rays utilized travel in the opposite direction to the cathode rays. In this way, a shorter focal tumour distance is retained and the inherent

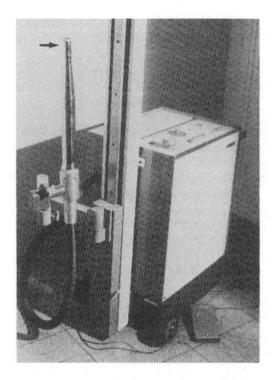

Fig. 10. Philips unit RT 50 used in intracavitary irradiation of rectal cancer. The X-ray tube is shown by the *arrow*

filtration of the tube is reduced. Its light weight compared to the SIEMENS machine makes it very easy for the operator to use.

The maximum energy is 50 kV. The X-ray tube has an extremely thin mica-beryllium window with an inherent filtration of 0.3 mm aluminium equivalency (Al) The tube is rod-shaped and air-cooled, and radiation is emitted axially from it. The shortest focal distance for skin tumour application is 2 cm. In the case of intrarectal application the focal distance is 4 cm, thanks to the use of a special applicator 29 mm in diameter (Fig. 11). Two extrafilters can be used: 0.5 mm Al, the most commonly used; and 1 mm Al. The output is 2000 R/min with the 0.5 mm Al filter, and 800 R/min with the 1 mm Al filter. These figures may surprise the radiotherapist accustomed to deep therapy. As was stressed by VAN DER PLAATS (1938), there is nothing terrifying in a superficial dose of 4000 R given in 2 min when it is realized that it is applied to morbid tissue, and when one is certain that in those layers where cells must be spared only a much lower dose is active. A high radiation output is of great practical importance, since it permits the radiation times to be appreciably curtailed. This machine produces a very inhomogeneous radiation, which decreases in depth so rapidly that the tissue-saving effect, which is the very aim of contact therapy, is manifested to a high degree. The depth exposure as percentage of the surface exposure is presented in Table 7.

By contrast with deep therapy, in the case of contact X-ray therapy at a certain depth the tissue can be regarded as practically undamaged and as fully capable of recuperative action. The surface of the field of irradiation is related to the treatment applicator; it is annular and measures 29 mm in diamter. In the

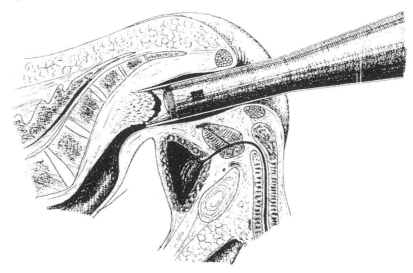

Fig. 11. Principle of intrarectal irradiation. The X-ray tube is introduced into the treatment applicator. The distance between the X-ray focus and the end of the tube is 4 cm. The rectal tumour is irradiated directly without interposition of soft tissue

Table 7. Percentage depth exposure with PHILIPS RT 50 machine (energy 50 kV, focal distance 4 cm)

Depth in water	Depth exposure as % of the skin exposure	
	Extrafilter 0.5 mm Al	Extrafilter 1 mm Al
0 mm	100%	100%
5 mm	44%	62%
10 mm	23%	38%
15 mm	14%	23%
20 mm	9%	15%
30 mm	4%	8%

case of two overlapping fields, the surface irradiated is 4.5 cm in length by 3 cm in width. The volume within which the radiation effect takes place is very small compared to that in other radiation technique. The high dose delivered at each application, which results in a rapid shrinkage of superficial layers of the exophytic part of the tumour, necessitates a treatment performed in a small number of applications separated by a free interval of 1, 2, or 3 weeks, the destruction of the tumour occurring layer by layer.

Intrarectal Applications. It must be noticed that the exposure dose in contact X-ray therapy is calculated in roentgens (R), whereas the absorbed dose in external irradiation or interstitial curietherapy is calculated in rads. In contact X-ray therapy applied to rectal tumours, because of the differences between superficial doses and deep doses, and the rapid shrinkage of the lesion, an exact absorbed dose cannot be calculated in rads, as it is in teletherapy. The dose which is applied in contact therapy is essentially based on clinical observation and determined

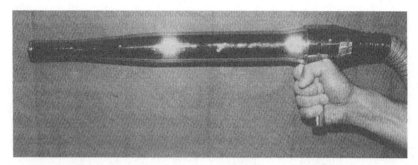

Fig. 12. Technique of free-hand shooting. The radiotherapist holds the X-ray tube by its handgrip and can handle it easily

according to the features of the tumour, and not before starting treatment. Practically the overall dose varies between 10 000 and 15 000 R.

Free-hand Shooting Technique (VAN DER PLAATS 1938). One of the most significant features of the Philips machine is the fact that the radiotherapist can hold the X-ray tube in his hand, the tube being removed from the stand of the machine (Fig. 12). The very short radiation time of the application and the practical tube construction allow the radiotherapist to "shoot" this radiation, holding the tube by its handgrip and aiming it as one would a pistol. For this radiation straight from the hand, the contact X-ray tube is fitted into the applicator.

This method of irradiation can be easily applied without any danger for the operator or the aides who attend the application. The X-ray shielding incorporated in the equipment amply meets international protection requirements. The predominantly soft radiation emitted by the X-ray tube minimizes the degree of backscatter. In the case of intrarectal applications, backscatter radiation at the handgrip of the tube has been measured under clinical conditions. For an exposure of 1 000 R at a kV/filter combination of 50 kV/0.5 mm Al, the intrarectal treatment applicator being held with the left hand and, shielded by the operator's leaded rubber glove, the dose delivered at the handgrip of the tube is 0.00007 R, or 0.07 mR. International Council for Radiological Protection (ICRP) recommendations state that the maximum yearly radiation exposure is 5 R per person. If the average dose delivered at each treatment is 3 000 R, from the foregoing worked example the maximum number of treatments per year that could be administered by one operator would be 25 000.

This suggests that intrarectal contact X-ray therapy may be practised without any danger to the operator and his assistants. It is recommended, however, that a leaded apron be worn whenever one is operating the equipment.

b) Interstitial Curietherapy

In oncology, curietherapy has a privileged place in the curative treatment of many malignant tumours, such as uterine cervix carcinomas and neoplasms of the oral cavity. However, curietherapy is only applicable to accessible tumours and to a well-defined limited volume of neoplastic tissue. Any attempt to control extensive tumours by curietherapy alone will result, in most cases, in failure and in severe radionecrotic complications. This is the reason why, in gynaecological or anal tumours, the present tendency is to combine external irradiation and curietherapy. External irradiation is used first, and aims at reducing the size of the tumour to a large extent. The purpose of the interstitial curietherapy is to deliver a booster dose to the central part of the tumour, which is considered less radiosensitive and in need of a higher dose of radiation, due to the presence of a large proportion of hypoxic cells.

Historically, radium and radon were the first sources of radiation successfully used to treat patients with small localized rectal cancers. The experience of BINKLEY reported in 1938 is exemplary in this respect. The protocol used by this author consisted of external irradiation for 3 weeks, and interstitial radium- or radon-therapy 2 weeks later. In a series of 65 cases there were 19 large, 28 medium, and 18 small tumours. Of the 19 patients with advanced disease, four enjoyed freedom from disease for a period of more than 5 years. Of the 28 cases treated for medium-sized tumours, 10 were alive and clinically disease-free. BINKLEY (1938) stressed that the most gratifying results concerned the 18 patients who had small tumours, but were considered to be high surgical risk: 15 of them were alive and well for periods varying from 15 months to 10 years. This experience is the most significant demonstration of the effectiveness of local irradiation of rectal cancer.

The statistics of the Mayo Clinic published by RUFF et al. (1961) are also very informative, since pre-operative radium implants were able to destroy rectal cancer locally in ten cases in a series of 96 patients treated by the same procedure.

However, since 1948 curietherapy for rectal tumours has been completely abandoned because of the important progress of surgery during the last 3 decades. Resectability rate and cure rate have been substantially improved, operative mortality rates have also significantly decreased, and during this entire period there have been very few publications regarding the role of curietherapy in the curative treatment of rectal cancers.

Nevertheless, many changes have occurred in curietherapy since 1960. Radium has been replaced by radioisotopes, in particular iridium-192. Compared with radium, the principal advantages of iridium-192 in interstitial curietherapy are:
1. Perfect parallelism and equidistance of radio-active sources
2. Length and activity of radioactive material chosen according to individual tumour
3. After-loading techniques consisting in using non-radioactive guides prior to placing the radioactive materials. The non-radioactive insertion is performed without any hurry, the guides being manipulated and adjusted with no radiation hazard. The parallelism of the non-radioactive application is controlled by X-ray films and image intensifier
4. Easy and accurate dosimetry.

These revolutionary changes have increased the homogeneity of irradiation and the efficacy of curietherapy, and made it not only less empirical but able to solve new clinical problems.

However, it is admitted that curietherapy remains a method of irradiation mainly applicable to limited, highly curable tumours, even if it can be of some help in cases of advanced tumours unsuitable for surgery as recently demonstrated by SYED (1975).

At the Southern California Cancer Center, SYED and FEDER (1971) and SYED et al. (1978) and JACKSON (1980) have initiated an after-loading programme of interstitial curietherapy applicable to primary or recurrent anorectal tumours. Iridium-192 is the isotope used:

The implant is performed in the operating room usually under regional or a light general anaesthesia. After careful examination of the tumour, the perianal skin is marked with an outline of the circumference of the template. A soft rubber rectal catheter is inserted. As the tumour is palpated the first thin (17-gauge) stainless steel needle is inserted through the perianal skin into the depths of the tumour. Next a careful engineered plastic inner template, tailored to the individual problem and ensuing uniform source distribution, is fitted over the needle and several more steel needles inserted. The outer template is put into place over the inserted needles and the remaining needles are installed. The needles are anchored in place in the templates by set screws at the circumference and the templates are held to the patient's skin with sutures.

After the patient's recovery from anaesthesia, dummy radio-active sources are threaded into the needles and the patient is X-rayed to demonstrate the distribution of the needles and sources. The dosimetry is then computerized and after the patient has returned to his room, afterloading with Iridium 192 is carried out. The Iridium is threaded into the steel needles and anchored to the needles with special stainless steel buttons. When the dosimetry is calculated, the exact dosage to the tumour is accomplished and the template, needles and Iridium are removed at the precise predetermined time. This period is usually 2 or 3 days.

These authors, in 1978, reported their experience in the management of ten advanced tumours treated by a combination of external irradiation (4000–5000 rad) and two implants delivering 2000 rad each separated by an interval of 2–3 weeks. These were eight rectal adenocarcinomas and two epidermoid anal cancers. Five of ten patients were alive and well, with an average follow-up period of 24 months. Four complications were observed: one necrosis and three severe proctitis. This experience is of some value, but the correct role of interstitial curietherapy is in the management of rectal cancers as a supplement to contact X-ray therapy.

An experience of intracavitary irradiation applied to recurrences after transanal tumour excision for rectal cancer was reported by KOZLOVA and POPOVA (1977) of Moscow, using a gamma-ray emitter of cobalt-60. Several sources were used, according to the site and size of the lesion. The sources introduced per anum were located in contact with the lesion; the dose rate was 80–100 rad/h at the mucosa and 40–50 rad at 1 cm depth. The dose given at each application was 400–500 rad, the total dose 5000–6000 rad. The application took place every other day. Out of 17 patients with recurrences after local excision, 12 were cured, whilst four were disease-free for 1–3 years, two for 4 years, and six for 5–10 years. KOZLOVA and POPOVA mentioned that during recent years they had used a new intracavitary irradiation unit called AGAT-V, which gave a dose rate of 20 rad/min and was more convenient than the previous one with regard to the treatment time.

Technique Used at the Centre Léon Bérard. The purpose of interstitial curietherapy is not to treat large tumours of the rectum; it is only used as a supplementary

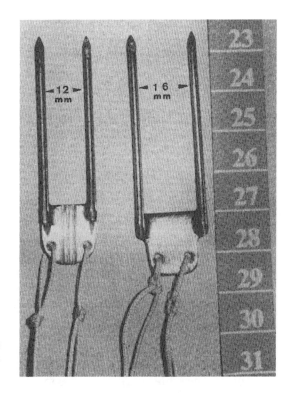

Fig. 13. Steel forks used for iridium-192 implant. They have two prongs 16 mm or 12 mm apart. Each prong is pre-loaded with an iridium wire 4 cm long

method after contact X-ray therapy and applied to give a booster dose to the bed of the tumour, i.e. to a very limited target volume in the rectal wall. Between 1951 and 1973, radium needles 4 cm long (3 cm active length) loaded with 4 mg radium were used. They were easily implanted in the rectal wall through a large rectoscope. Three to four radium needles were inserted 1 cm apart, but the parallelism of the needles and the homogeneity of the irradiation were never satisfactory. This is the reason why radium needles have been replaced by two wires of iridium-192 in a fork since 1979.

At present, the material used is a rigid steel fork with two straight hollow prongs, 4 cm long, pointed at the free end, the tip of each prong obturated by a spot of welding. The two prongs, 16 mm or 12 mm apart, are welded to a base-plate (Fig. 13). There are two holes in the base-plate in which two threads are fixed which will be used for the withdrawal of the fork. Each prong is pre-loaded with an iridium-192 wire 4 cm long. The curietherapy is carried out 6 weeks after completion of contact X-ray therapy, the tumour being abraded. The purpose of implantation is to increase the chance of local control.

Curietherapy does not require anaesthesia, general or local. The patient is placed in the knee-chest position. The 29-mm PHILIPS applicator is introduced through the anus so that the operator gets a clear view of the site of the bed of the growth. The fork is firmly held by special forceps, then introduced into the lumen of the rectoscope and implanted in the rectal wall at a distance of 1 cm below the site of the area to be treated. It is easily inserted upwards, almost parallel to the

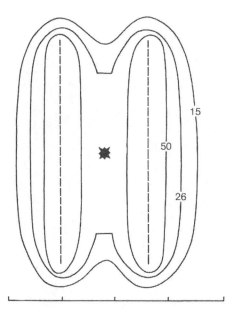

Fig. 14. Isodose distribution in frontal plane of the 16-mm iridium fork. A dose of 26 rad/h for 1 mCi/cm is delivered on the reference isodose curve. Intervals of 1 cm are indicated below the diagram

axis of the rectal ampulla. The iridium fork is not sutured to the rectal wall. A rubber drain enveloped in greasy gauze pushed through the anus is used to keep the fork in place. The rubber drain is sutured to the skin of the anal margin under local anaesthesia. After the treatment time has elapsed, the stitch which fixed the rubber drain is cut, and the iridium fork is then easily removed, together with the rubber drain, by pulling the wires fixed to the base-plate of the fork. Anaesthesia is not required. The dose delivered is 2000 to 3000 rad. Very active iridium wires are used (4–6 mCi/cm). The treatment time does not exceed 24 h and immediate tolerance is excellent, in most cases.

Dosimetric Control. Dosimetry determines the effective distribution of the dose. Two methods of control are used: direct dosimetry via a detector placed in vivo, and indirect dosimetry using the computer. With direct dosimetry, the detector of a SIEMENS gamma meter is introduced into the rectum immediately after insertion of the iridium fork, and the detector is placed on the rectal mucosa in several places in the irradiated volume: in the centre of the treated area, i.e. between the two radioactive lines, at the level of the tip of the fork; and around its base-plate. A homogeneous dose is delivered between the two prongs, whereas rapid fluctuations of dose are measured beside the prongs. With indirect dosimetry, two orthogonal X-ray films of the pelvic area are taken. A constant magnification factor of 0.33 is used. X-ray films check the parallelism of the two radioactive lines. Computer dosimetry gives a clear idea of the irradiated target volume, with the isodose curves drawn in several planes (Fig. 14). With two straight iridium wires, parallel, 16 mm apart, 4 cm long, and a lineic activity of 1 mCi/cm, a dose of 26 rad/h is delivered in a target volume 3.5 cm long, 2.5 cm large, and 1.3 cm wide. With the two wires 12 mm apart the dose is 34 rad/h.

Sometimes a slight convergence of the free ends of the prongs alters the dose distribution. In such cases, a reconstruction of the geometric configuration can be made, which determines the basal dose and the 85% references isodose according to the Paris dosimetric method, described by PIERQUIN et al. (1978). This is used for the calculation of the time, in correlation with the lineic activity of the two wires.

c) Development of Intracavitary Irradiation

In 1946, LAMARQUE and GROS, Montpellier, France, with great shrewdness, recognized the possibility of applying the contact X-ray tube built by PHILIPS to the management of cancer of the rectum. They were the true pioneers of the present technique of intracavitary irradiation of rectal cancer, and drew up the guidelines for the practice of this method. They used to give a dose of 1 800–2 000 R per application up to a total dose of between 15 000 and 30 000 R. They stressed the advantage of delivering a higher dose at the first application and using a filter of 1 mm Al for the last treatment instead of 0.5 mm Al for the first treatments.

The overall treatment time was 2–3 months, and they emphasized the necessity of using the time factor to assess the shrinkage of the tumour, and of adapting the dose and the focalization to the clinical findings at every sitting.

They conducted a study of the histological changes which occur after contact X-ray therapy in the neoplastic tissue, as well as in the underlying structures of the rectal wall. They observed early signs of cytoplasmic and nuclear degeneration which started a few hours after the treatment and increased during the few days following. They showed that bowel epithelium was destroyed by a single dose of 4 000 R, but that regeneration was completed 1 month later. They noticed the high resistance of the muscular layers of the rectal wall, which are not seriously altered at these treatment doses, and the absence of perforation under the conditions of intrarectal contact X-ray therapy. They reported on a series of 116 patients with cancer of the rectum treated by contact X-ray therapy in an experimental way: 70% of tumours were advanced, inoperable lesions (group III); 17% were large, still movable cancers (group II); and only 23% were limited and freely mobile tumours (group I). The cure rates at 5 years are shown in Table 8.

Interpretation of the cure rates reported by LAMARQUE and GROS must take into consideration the fact that there had been no previous work of this type. The rules for selection of tumours suitable for conservative treatment were not yet known, nor were the relationships between the probability of lymphatic spread and local spread and histological degree of differentiation. The relatively modest results obtained in the treatment of limited tumours (group 1) are explained by

Table 8. Five-year survival rates following contact X-ray therapy (Lamarque and Gros 1954)

Classification	No. of cases	5-year survival rate
Group I	26	42%
Group II	20	30%
Group III	70	20%

the fact that most patients referred to LAMARQUE and GROS were poor risk or inoperable.

It must also be remembered that the publications of LAMARQUE and GROS (1946, 1954), as well as those of CHAOUL and WACHSMANN (1953), aroused distrust, both because the intracavitary irradiation of rectal tumours was a revolutionary technique, the principles of which were completely opposed to those of the conventional X-ray therapy, and because adenocarcinoma of the rectum was considered to be radioresistant, and it seemed inconceivable that irradiation could control such a lesion.

The most important contribution of LAMARQUE and GROS was not merely the introduction to medical practice of a new method of local treatment of rectal cancer, but above all the definition of the rules for selection of cases suitable for such irradiation, and the attempt to convince the medical world of the contribution of this method in the management of early rectal cancer.

In the following years, small series of rectal cancer treated according to LARMARQUE's method were reported by RUCKENSTEINER (1954, 14 of 18 patients cured), and by VILLACEQUE et al. at the Institut Gustave Roussy, Paris (1962, 9 patients out of 13 cured; the failures were related in 2 cases to wrong selection, in 1 case to a local and nodal recurrence; there was one indeterminate death), and by GONDARD (1951, 2 patients out of 3 were cured; the only failure was related to a metastatic lymph node in the mesorectum, treated by AP resection).

PARTURIER-ALBOT (1965, 1979), in a long series of publications, reported on 318 cases of limited rectal cancer treated by contact X-ray therapy alone or by contact X-ray therapy followed by local excision of the irradiated area with 96% of long-term local control.

In 1980, SISCHY and REMINGTON (1975, 1976) and SISCHY et al. (1978, 1980 a, b, c; Highland Hospital, Rochester, New York) reported a large series of limited rectal carcinoma treated by contact X-ray therapy in the United States. The technique of irradiation and the selection of the cases were similar to that applied at the Centre Léon Bérard. Their experience included 74 patients treated radically and 31 treated palliatively. They described four cases who were rejected for treatment because of palpable nodes and confirmed that these nodes were usually felt immediately cephalic to the lesion at a distance of 2–3 cm. Shrinkage of the tumours was so rapid that by the third treatment visualization of the original lesion was often difficult.

Of 74 patients treated for cure since 1973, only four patients had local failures of treatment; one of them had a poorly differentiated adenocarcinoma which was not considered to be suitable for conservative therapy. Eleven patients had died from other causes. The absence of local failure had been confirmed at postmortem. Seventy patients followed up for at least 18 months were alive and well and disease-free (94%).

In the series of 31 patients treated only palliatively by contact X-ray therapy and in some cases subsequently by radium needling (2 500 R), SISCHY was able to obtain a good local control in 69% of cases. This interesting series stressed the close collaboration that must exist between radiotherapist and surgeon.

JELDEN et al. (1981), at the Cleveland Clinic, applied intracavitary radiation therapy with the PHILIPS unit as definitive treatment to 44 patients with limited rectal adenocarcinoma. Thirty-seven patients had no evidence of disease up to 85 months, three died of intercurrent disease and four were treatment failures. Of the four failures, three were free of disease at the primary site after subsequent surgery.

d) Experience at the Centre Léon Bérard (PAPILLON 1968, 1973, 1974, 1975a, b, c; 1977, 1979, 1980a, b; 1981) and PAPILLON and BAILLY (1979)

Technique. Contact X-ray therapy with the PHILIPS machine has been applied to rectal tumours in Lyon since 1951. LAMARQUE's method has been adopted from general principles and progressively modified according to the information drawn from successes and, even more importantly, failures, carefully observed. Simultaneously, interstitial curietherapy has been introduced as an additional technique to extend the range of indications for intracavitary irradiation. The principles of this method are essentially different from those generally used in radiation oncology. This work has always been carried out in close collaboration with surgeons, gastro-enterologists, and proctologists.

At the time of decision, the radiotherapist must be fully aware that the purpose of intracavitary irradiation is the cure of the patient by control of his tumour. Any failure can jeopardize the life of the patient, and the radiotherapist therefore carries a heavy responsibility.

Before starting intrarectal contact X-ray therapy the radiotherapist should determine with great accuracy the microscopical and gross features of the lesion, paying attention to the following details:

1. Histological grade of malignancy, studied on several biopsies. High-grade tumours are not suitable.
2. Level of the lower and upper edges of the growth from the anal verge; circumferential extent and quadrants involved; consistency; configuration of the cancer: polypoid, slightly or greatly protruding into the rectal lumen, ulcerative, erosive, disc-like; degree of infiltration of the rectal wall; mobility of the tumour on the rectal wall; mobility of the rectal wall in the invaded area; width and thickness of the growth.
3. Integrity of the surrounding rectal wall, especially above the primary tumour; absence of palpable lymph node.
4. Perfect accessibility to the whole tumour and particularly to upper edge of the lesion in the lumen of the 29-mm applicator.

If these findings, carefully determined, comply with the criteria of selection for conservative treatment, contact X-ray therapy represents a suitable alternative method of treatment.

The treatment is performed in the out-patient department and does not require admission to hospital. Between each application, the patient can have a normal active life. After cleansing the rectum with a Microlax, the patient is placed in the knee-chest position on the rectoscopy couch, the head turned to the right, the left cheek lying directly on the couch, the back hollowed. Some elderly or handicapped patients may be unable to hollow their back: the couch is then inclined to an angle of 20°–30°. In this way the position of the trunk permits the

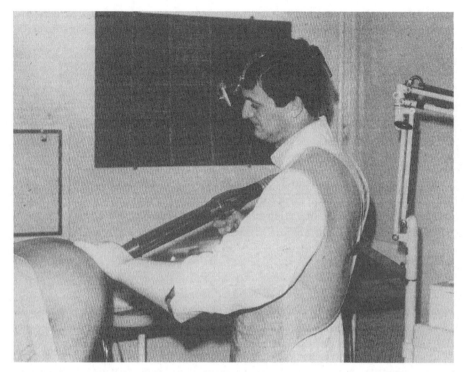

Fig. 15. During the treatment the operator has a forehead lamp and wears a leaded rubber apron and a leaded rubber left glove. The X-ray tube held by his right hand is fitted in the treatment applicator, which is firmly held by his left hand

contents of the pelvis to fall upwards into the abdominal cavity and the walls of the rectum fall apart, opening the rectal lumen.

The operator introduces his right index finger to relax the anal sphincter. Then, using Xylocaine Gel (lidocaine) as a lubricant, he introduces the 24-mm rectoscope, which begins to dilate the anal canal; a little later this is exchanged for the 29-mm treatment applicator.[1] The careful and slow introduction of this larger tube does not generally require anaesthesia. However, in patients with narrowing of the anal canal, or spasm or tenderness of the anus, local anaesthesia with lidocaine (2%) may be needed before the first application. In general in such patients, anaesthesia is not necessary for subsequent treatments. Then the obturator of the rectoscope is withdrawn.

The radiotherapist, if he wishes, wears a leaded rubber apron and a leaded rubber left glove (Fig. 15). With the aid of a forehead lamp or a cold light device, he checks the position of the tumour in the lumen of the treatment applicator, holding the latter firmly with his left hand. With the tip of the applicator, the radiotherapist applies pressure on the rectal wall near the lower edge of the tumour,

---

[1] Treatment applicators of several types are built by Arplay Inc., Izeure 21110, France.

so that the lesion presents in the axis of the applicator, the end of the applicator being applied to the invaded area. This pressure is the best method of delivering a fairly homogeneous dose of radiation to the surface of the tumour. The left hand is steadied by resting on the left buttock of the patient. This guides and maintains the position of the treatment applicator, which defines the field of irradiation.

Then the X-ray tube, held by the handgrip in the right hand of the operator, is fitted in the treatment applicator, without changing the position of the left hand. Everything is ready for the first application. The apparatus is switched on by pressing the footswitch to start. When irradiation is emitted, an indicator lamp lights and a warning buzzer sounds. When the irradiation time setting has elapsed, radiation is automatically switched off and the lamp and the buzzer are deactivated.

The X-ray tube works at 50 kV. Extrafilter 0.5 mm Al is used for the first applications. Extrafilter 1 mm Al is used for the last treatment applied on the bed of the tumour. Each application lasts 1–3 min.

During the application, the operator must insist on the complete immobility of the patient. At any given time, the treatment can be interrupted and the X-ray tube withdrawn, if it is desired to check (by sighting through the applicator) whether the correct position of the field of irradiation is being maintained. If the tumour is polypoid and very protruding, the lesion can be invaginated into the applicator. In such cases, the dose given to the surface of the tumour is much higher than the calculated dose, because of the decrease in the focal distance. In each case, the time of the application is interrupted two or three times to check the position of the field, for instance, every 30 s.

If the size of the tumour exceeds the size of the end of the applicator, it is necessary to use, for the first applications, two overlapping fields, an upper and a lower. The surface covered by the two fields is 4.5 cm long by 2.9 cm wide. When using two overlapping fields, no serious complications need be feared due to local necrosis or delay of healing. The overdosage related to the overlapping is limited to a small volume of the tumour in its central part, which in any case requires the highest dose of radiation.

The whole treatment consists of four to five applications, over a period of 6–8 weeks. The second applications is made 1 or 2 weeks after the first, on day 8 or 15; the third on day 21 or 28; the fourth, and generally the last, on day 42 or 49. Rarely a fifth application is needed a few weeks later. The dose given at each application varies from 2000 R to 4000 R on one field. The total dose per field does not exceed 10000–14000 R.

The characteristics of intrarectal contact X-ray therapy may be summarized as follows: High doses of superficially penetrating radiations directly applied to the tumour on limited surfaces, the field being circular, 29 mm in diameter. The treatment is given in a small number of applications (usually four over a period of 6–8 weeks, with long intervals between treatments).

These special conditions of irradiation explain the particular effectiveness of the method. High doses given at every treatment produce a rapid shrinkage of the exophytic part of the tumour. Hence at the second application on day 8, a week after the first, the tumour usually has a greatly reduced volume compared with its initial size. The same process is noticed at subsequent applications.

The tumour is destroyed layer by layer; each application treats a different layer of the tumour from the previous one. Before the second, third, and fourth applications, all changes in the appearance of the lesion are carefully noted in the case report.

The rapid shrinkage of the lesion is a proof of the high radiosensitivity of limited rectal adenocarcinoma treated by intracavitary irradiation. The reduction in size affects both the width and the thickness of the lesion. The diameter of the invaded area of the rectal mucosa decreases significantly between day 1 and day 21, so that in the case of rather large tumours – 4–5 cm in diameter – irradiated initially via two fields, only one field is needed from the third application. The reduction in thickness of the tumour varies according to the configuration of the lesion. In the case of exophytic cancers, largely protruding into the rectal lumen, the thickness decreases significantly after day 8. Conversely, in the case of more infiltrating lesions, ulcerative or disc-like, the reduction in thickness of the tumour is slower. The rapidity of the shrinkage is used as a guideline at each treatment to define the dose to be given and the interval before the next application.

Endoscopic examination shows that during the period of treatment the rectal cancer is brought back to its point of origin, with gradual regression of tumour bulk, each tumour maintaining its particular shape. Thus a large polypoid cancer becomes a small polypoid cancer before total destruction of the tumour. The same process is observed in the case of ulcerative tumours.

For cases of ulcerative or more infiltrating tumours still confined to the rectal wall, doubt may exist about the control of the bed of the tumour, i.e. the area of involvement within the rectal wall. In such cases, interstitial curietherapy is needed.

Bleeding, which is the most common symptom of rectal cancer, usually stops a few days after the first application. This improvement corresponds to the rapid shrinkage of the exophytic portion of the tumour. During the treatment, diet and daily routine are entirely normal.

The excellent tolerance of intracavitary contact X-ray therapy is related to the protection of the rectal wall during the first part of the treatment. At the first and second applications, the dose is almost exclusively concentrated on the tumour, and the rectal wall is completely spared. At the third and fourth applications, the

---

Plate 3

Fig. III. A. Well differentiated polypoid adenocarcinoma of the posterior part of the rectum, before treatment.

Fig. III. B. After 4 applications of Contact X-ray therapy. The scar is almost invisible. The tumor has entirely disappeared. There is normal suppleness of rectal wall in the irradiated area.

Fig. IV. A. Well differentiated polypoid adenocarcinoma before treatment.

Fig. IV. B. The same one week later after one application of Contact X-ray therapy (4000 R). The shrinkage is striking.

Fig. IV. C. The same after completion of Contact X-ray therapy. Rectal mucosa almost normal.

Intracavitary Irradiation of Rectal Tumours

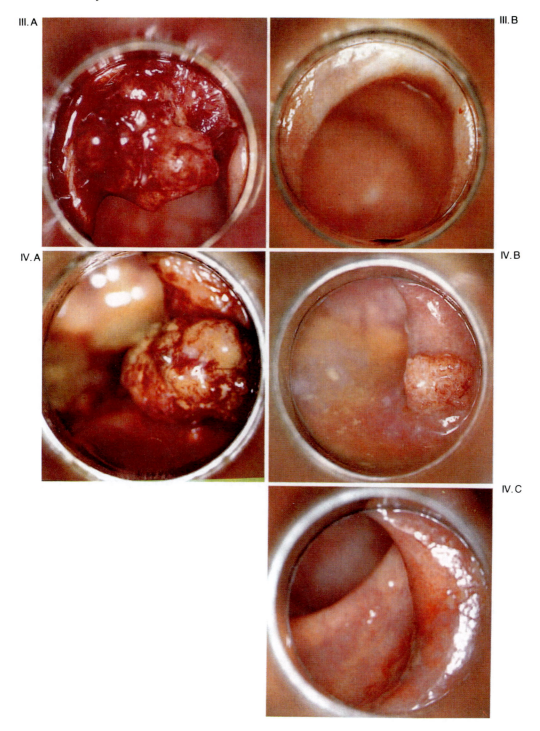

III. A III. B
IV. A IV. B
IV. C

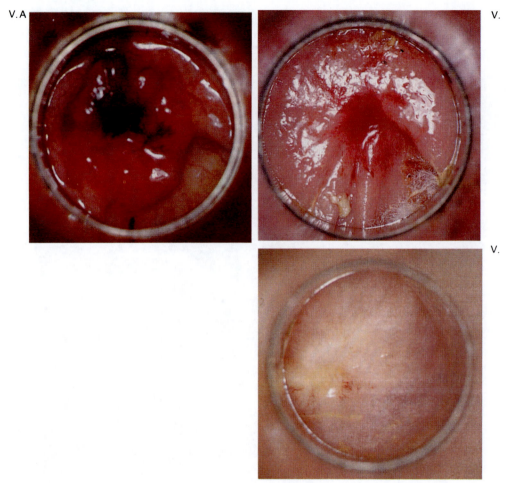

Plate 4

Fig. V. A. Ulcerative and bulky adenocarcinoma, 2.5 cm in diameter, in a 70-year old woman, before treatment.

Fig. V. B. The same, five weeks later after 4 applications of Contact X-ray therapy (total exposure 14000 R). Central ulceration remains, before curietherapy.

Fig. V. C. Final result after curietherapy. A trophic appearance of the mucosa. No stricture of the rectal lumen. The rectal wall remains perfectly supple. The patient is well after more than twelve years.

rectal wall is necessarily irradiated, but the doses given are within the limits of the tolerance. In the case of small tumours, 2 cm or less in diameter, it is possible to use for the last two treatments a special applicator 24 mm in diameter, in order to protect the surrounding normal rectal wall.

When the irradiation treatment is finished, many patients do not have any local reaction. Some have a very slight proctitis, which does not last more than 2 or 3 weeks. Radionecrosis is rare (8%). Some are asymptomatic, some painful, They are always superficial and do not last more than 1 month.

A question may be raised: *Why does a cancer known to be radioresitant or only slightly radiosensitive become highly radiosensitive and radiocurable when treated by intracavitary contact X-ray therapy?*

The favourable, and maybe unexpected, response of limited rectal adenocarcinomas to contact X-ray therapy is related to an important difference between time-dose and volume-dose relationships in contact X-ray therapy and in external cobalt therapy. With external supervoltage irradiation, a dose of 4000 rad is given over 4 weeks to a very large volume of normal tissue. With contact X-ray therapy, a dose of 4000 R is delivered in 2 min to a very small volume of tissue. This is the explanation of the particular effectiveness of this type of irradiation applied to limited rectal cancers.

In conclusion, contact X-ray therapy is the principal method of intracavitary irradiation of rectal cancer for cure. In all cases, this method is used first, and in most cases it results in a control of those exophytic tumours which are confined to the rectal wall.

Results. Two hundred and eighty patients with limited rectal cancer have been treated by intracavitary irradiation since 1951. During this period there have been several changes. In the first 10 years, most tumours treated with curative intent were limited and polypoid, and the treatment consisted exclusively of contact X-ray therapy. Since 1960 more ulcerative cancers have been treated and interstitial curietherapy has played a greater part as a supplement following contact therapy. During the first years curietherapy was performed with radium needles. They were replaced by the iridium-192 fork in 1972. Such developments were a response to wider indications for intracavitary irradiation, although patients were still carefully selected for this procedure.

After the first 10 years criteria for selection became more precise, with an increase in the number of cases suitable for local treatment. A search for palpable metastatic nodes has been made routinely since 1968. During the past 13 years the selection of those ulcerative carcinomas has been improved by assessment of their response to treatment over 3 weeks. Finally, a technique of mesenteric and perirectal lymphadenectomy has been used for selected patients since 1971.

The following statistics are concerned with all the cases which seemed suitable for intracavitary irradiation.

All tumours were true invasive carcinomas with the exclusion of: in situ carcinomas, cancers in polyps, and malignant change in villous adenomas.

All tumours were well – or moderately well – differentiated adenocarcinomas on multiple biopsies. Grade III and IV poorly differentiated carcinomas, as well as colloid carcinomas, were excluded because of the high probability of regional spread.

Rectal cancers associated with familial polyposis previously treated by total colectomy and ileorectal anastomosis were excluded, as were synchronous colonic and rectal cancers. Three patients with such disease (not included in the figures) underwent resection for the lesion of the colon and irradiation for the rectal tumour. All three have remained alive and well for more than 5 years without recurrence.

All patients with ulcerative or infiltrating cancers who were thought to have local spread beyond the limits of the rectal wall at 3 weeks after two applications of contact X-ray therapy were referred for radical excision.

Approximately half the patients were poor surgical risks, either because of their age or because of poor general condition with associated disease. The average age was 62, the extremes being 25 and 88. Almost 38% of the patients were over 70, with 24% over 75.

Before starting intracavitary irradiation patients underwent a full clinical examination and a barium enema to exclude a synchronous lesion of the large bowel. Where there was doubt about the status of the liver, scintigraphy, or more recently EMI scanning, was performed. The CEA level has also been measured during the last few years.

Two hundred and sixty tumours (93%) were within reach of the examining finger in the distal 9 cm of the large bowel. Adenocarcinomas of the anal and juxta-anal area are not included in this series; they will be analysed on p. 95.

Two hundred and seven cases have been followed for more than 5 years; 150 (72.5%) tumours were not larger than 3 cm in diameter and were therefore treated by only one field of contact X-ray therapy in most cases. Fifty-seven (27.5%) tumours exceeded 3 cm, and were treated by two overlapping fields of contact X-ray therapy during the first applications.

One hundred and fifty-eight (76.3%) were essentially protuberant or polypoid, with little evidence of infiltration. Forty-nine (23.6%) were ulcerative and

---

Plate 5

Fig. VI. A. Ulcerative and vegetating adenocarcinoma, 4.5 cm in length, in a 74-year old man, before treatment.

Fig. VI. B. The same after contact X-ray therapy and Radium implant. The patient is well more than eight years later.

Fig. VII. A. Ulcerative adenocarcinoma (4 cm in diameter) in a 82-year old patient, before treatment.

Fig. VII. B. The same after contact X-ray therapy (two overlapping fields) and Iridium implant. The rectal wall appears completely normal. Patient alive and well six years after treatment.

Fig. VIII. A. Ulcerative and excavated adenocarcinoma in a 83-year old patient, before treatment.

Fig. VIII. B. The same after contact X-ray therapy (4 applications). Note the telangiectasia of the mucosa. No bleeding. The patient died 7 years later from intercurrent disease. No recurrence. He was 90 years old.

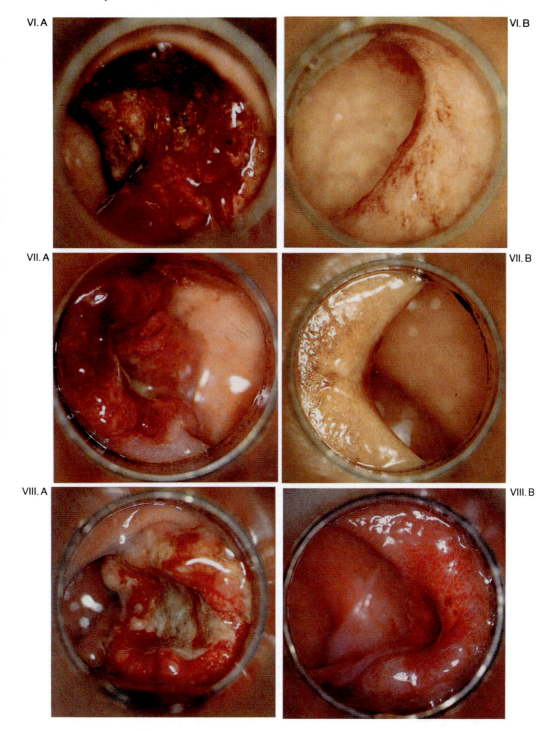

more infiltrating adenocarcinomas. The percentage of combined treatment (contact + curietherapy) as compared with contact X-Ray therapy alone was 20% before 1965, whereas it is at present 50%.

Before starting treatment the procedure was explained to the patients. The importance of cooperation with the radiotherapist and the need for long-term follow-up for many years after completion of the irradiation were both stressed. Approximately one-quarter of the patients were referred by surgeons, and three-quarters by proctologists or gastro-enterologists.

Of the 207 patients followed up for over 5 years (Table 9), 153 are alive and well with no evidence of disease. The 5-year survival rate is 73.9%. (One hundred and forty-five have been cured by irradiation alone and a further eight have been salvaged by surgery after irradiation failed to cure them. Five of these eight patients had a radical excision with a permanent colostomy, and three had a conservative procedure without bowel section (one anterior resection, two perirectal lymphadenectomies). Normal sphincter control of intestinal function has been conserved in 148 of the 153 cured patients.

Fifty-four patients died, 28 (13.5%) from intercurrent disease or a second primary cancer. Four died post-operatively after AP resection, either for failure (two), or for indurated scar, erroneously considered as local failure (two) in disagreement with the opinion of the radiotherapist. Some patients who were still alive with cancer treated palliatively at the end of the 5th year are included among the 22 patients (10.6%) considered as dead from cancer at 5 years; these patients died during the 6th year of follow-up.

There is a relationship between the size of the tumour and the chance of cure after conservative treatment by irradiation (Table 10). The 5-year survival rate is 80% for lesions 3 cm or less in diameter, whereas it is only 61.5% for tumours larger than 3 cm. The rates of death from cancer are 6% and 22.8% respectively.

The configuration of the tumour seems to have less prognostic significance than the size of the lesion (Table 11). The 5-year survival rates are not statistically different for polypoid and ulcerative tumours, as well as the rates of death from cancer. However, distant metastases occurred twice as frequently following ulcerative tumours.

One hundred and forty-six patients have been followed up for more than 10 years (Table 12). No recurrence or distant metastasis occurred between the 5th

Table 9. Intracavitary irradiation for cure of limited rectal cancers: Results at 5 years[a]

	No. of cases	Percentage
Patients treated	207	100
Alive and well more than 5 years	153	73.9
Deaths	54	26.1
Death from cancer	22	10.6
Death from intercurrent disease	28	13.5
Post-operative death	4	2
Local failures	11	5.3
Nodal failures	12	5.8
Distant metastasis	6	2.9

[a] Centre Léon Bérard.

Table 10. Intracavitary irradiation for cure of limited rectal cancers: Relationship between results and size of tumour in 207 cases[a]

	Tumours ≤ 3 cm	Tumours > 3 cm
Patients treated	150 (72.5%)	57 (27.5%)
5-year survival	120 (80%)	33 (57.8%)
Alive with normal anal function	117 (78%)	31 (54.3%)
Death from cancer	9 (6%)	13 (22.8%)
Death from interc. disease	19 (12.5%)	9 (15.7%)
Post-operative death	2 (1.3%)	2 (3.5%)
Local failures	7 (4.6%)	4 (7%)
Nodal failures	6 (4%)	6 (10.5%)
Distant metastases	3 (2%)	4 (7%)

[a] Centre Léon Bérard.

Table 11. Intracavitary irradiation for cure of limited rectal cancers: Relationship between results and configuration of tumour in 207 cases[a]

	Protuberant or polypoid tumour	Ulcerative tumour
No. of cases	158 (76.3%)	49 (23.6%)
5-year survival	115 (72.8%)	34 (69.3%)
Alive after subsequent surgery	4 (2.5%)	4 (8.1%)
Deaths from cancer	16 (10.1%)	6 (12.2%)
Deaths from interc. disease	23 (14.3%)	5 (10.2%)
Post-operative deaths	2 (1.2%)	2 (1.2%)
Local failures	6 (3.8%)	5 (10.2%)
Nodal failures	7 (4.4%)	5 (10.2%)

[a] Centre Léon Bérard.

Table 12. Intracavitary irradiation of rectal cancers: Results at 10 years[a]

	No. of cases
Patients treated	146
Alive and well at 10 years	85 (58%)
Deaths from cancer	14 (10%)
Deaths from intercurrent disease	43 (29.4%)
Post-operative deaths	4

[a] Centre Léon Bérard.

and the 10th years. Eighty-five patients (58%) were alive and well at over 10 years. Of the 61 patients who died, 14 (10%) died of rectal cancer, 12 of them before 5 years; two were alive at 5 years but with cancer and died during the 6th year. Four patients died post-operatively and 43 (29.4%) died of intercurrent disease without evidence of rectal cancer. In this series, no patients were lost to follow-up, and the causes of death were known in all cases. These figures show that after irradiation of limited rectal cancer, patients who are free from recurrence at 5 years can be considered to be cured.

Follow-up After Intracavitary Irradiation. Early detection of recurrence is the objective of follow-up after conservative treatment of cancer, irrespective of the site of the tumour and the therapeutic procedure. This deserves special attention in the case of rectal cancer because subsequent radical surgery may control local or nodal failures in many cases. It implies a careful and regular follow-up by the radiotherapist who has been in charge of the treatment. He knows the patient better than anyone else and is in the best position to assess the features of the tumour before and during irradiation, its size, its consistency, its thickness, and its degree of infiltration of the rectal wall. He will remember the stages of shrinkage of the lesion and will have assessed the appearance of the treated area at the end of the irradiation. Follow-up examination should take place every 2 months for the 1st year, every 3 months for the 2nd year, every 4 months for the 3rd year, every 6 months for the 4th and 5th years, and once a year after the 5th year. It is a demanding but reliable policy.

The aim of follow-up is the detection of local failures and the discovery of nodal failures, in the case of low-lying tumours, as well as distant metastases. Follow-up examination comprises general examination, chest X-ray, palpation of the liver, and CT scan of the liver in case of doubt. The dosage of CEA has not proved helpful in case of small rectal cancer. It can be done once a year. Double contrast enema or colonoscopy is needed every 2 years to exclude a metachronous carcinoma or polyp. Follow-up checking consists of (a) digital, (b) endoscopic, and sometimes, according to necessity, (3) cytological examination of scrape smears of the scar. This examination must be performed with the patient in the knee-chest position.

During the first weeks after intracavitary irradiation there is local inflammation of the treated area. The rectal mucosa is dark purple and bleeds easily on contact. Two months after the last session for polypoid cancers, the rectal mucosa has undergone regeneration and the rectal wall resumes a normal consistency without fibrosis. A few months later, the irradiated area can hardly be recognized except that it may be paler than the surrounding mucosa. After treatment of a more infiltrating lesion requiring higher doses to the bed of the tumour, especially if two overlapping fields have been needed, or if an iridium implant has been applied, a degree of ulceration will be found, often associated with symptoms of proctitis. This ulceration will heal quickly before the end of 3 months, and the mucosa will regenerate with telangiectasia and a little fibrosis of the underlying tissue. In a few cases, after the treatment of ulcerative tumours, a necrotic ulcer, which may be asymptomatic, may be noted for up to 4 months. A scrape smear may be needed to make sure that the lesion has been controlled. This ulceration will heal spontaneously or with steroid enemas.

Intracavitary irradiation never gives rise to stricture or narrowing of the rectal lumen, which keeps its normal size, making digital examination particularly easy at subsequent visits. During the follow-up period, 1 or 2 years after treatment, occasional bleeding may alarm patients. These episodes are related to the telangiectasia, and are easily controlled by local applications of dilute chromic acid 1:3. Digital examination will allow the radiotherapist to appreciate the consistency of the treated area, as compared with that of the adjacent rectal wall. Any change in consistency is noted on the case report. Three types of failure may be detected by follow-up examination: (a) distant metastasis without pelvic recurrence, (b) local failures in the treated area, (c) nodal failures in the mesorectum above the treated area.

Distant Metastases. Seven cases of distant metastasis to the liver or lung were observed in the series of 207 cases followed up over 5 years. One occurred in the 1st year, one in the 2nd year, one in the 3rd year, and four in the 4th year. No metastases were encountered after the 5th year. Distant metastases were observed twice as often in ulcerative tumours as in polypoid lesions, and more than three times as often in tumours larger than 3 cm as in smaller lesions. These failures cannot be attributed to the conservative method of treatment, but to the higher grade of malignancy of the disease submitted to irradiation, for they were observed in patients with cancer locally controlled by intrarectal irradiation.

Local Failures. Local failures may present in three ways: (a) the most common is an induration or a hard nodule in the rectal wall, under a normal or slightly atrophic mucosa; (b) an ulceration with a hardening at the centre of the lesion; (c) a proliferative lesion at the edge of the irradiated area. This latter presentation is quite rare. Its nature is easily proved by biopsy. In the case of a hard nodule covered by a healed mucosa, only transrectal biopsy performed per anum under general anaesthesia should demonstrate the failure, but clinical examination of the treated area performed by the radiotherapist himself is sufficient in most cases to decide on the need for further treatment by surgery. In cases of ulcerative abnormality of the rectal wall, a simple scrape smear for cytological investigation is a reliable measure. *The place of cytology in the follow-up must be stressed.*

The value and precision of cervicovaginal smears is abundantly clear, and WEBB (1979) has emphasized that it is surprising that a similar assessment of anorectal lesions has received little attention. He has published a series of 58 patients with anorectal or rectosigmoid disease, studied by a simple digital smear at rectal examination, or occasionally by scrape smear. Adequate smears were obtained in all cases; ten of them were normal controls. Forty-five of the lesions were histologically confirmed. The range of pathology included carcinoma of the rectum (19) and rectosigmoid (seven), anus (four), and villous papilloma (seven). There were 40 tumours, 31 of which were malignant. Positive identification of the neoplasm was made in 39 out of 40 cases (97%), with one suspect reading. There were no false positive reports and in three cases (7%) the initial histological biopsy was falsely negative.

At the Centre Léon Bérard, cytological survey of patients treated by intracavitary irradiation has been used during the follow-up period for the past 5 years. An adequate specimen is easily obtained by scraping with a wooden spatula the rectal mucosa in the treated area. Ethanol fixation and PAPANICOLAOU staining is employed.

In the rectum, normal smears contain columnar cells of rectal origin, some of them goblet cells. Cells are arranged either in a palisade pattern or in non-stratified sheets. The background is usually free of inflammation and necrosis. Faecal contamination is not important. In pathological smears, adenocarcinoma cells may be arranged in clusters of variable size, sometimes with lumen formation, on a bloody and necrotic background. Nuclear overlapping is always present. Isolated malignant cells may also appear. Cytoplasmic outlines are not clear. Nuclei are large, more or less hyperchromatic, and frequently nucleolated. After intracavitary irradiation, megalocytosis and typical nuclear alterations are considered as treatment-induced changes in normal as well as in malignant cells. It may be difficult to decide if the latter are viable. Another difficulty may be represented by "benign cellular atypies" and changes due to tissue repair. In such cases, cells are usually organized in sheets. These problems emphasize the need for clinical information by the cytopathologist and a close collaboration between the radiotherapist and the cytologist.

The experience at the Centre Léon Bérard is based on the study of 42 patients with rectal adenocarcinoma treated by intracavitary irradiation and checked by scrape smears during the follow-up period. A hundred smears were examined. In five cases material was inadequate and 95 evaluable smears were studied. There were positive smears in 25 cases, negative smears in 61 cases, and benign atypies in nine cases.

Correlation between cytology and biopsy pathology was possible in 13 cases. The small number of correlated cases is due to the reliability of cytology, which often makes biopsy unnecessary during the follow-up period. In ten cases there was a good correlation between the results of both methods (four negative, six positive). In three cases there was a discordance. In two cases cytology was negative, pathology positive. One of them can be explained by the deep location of the malignant proliferation in the rectal wall, whereas the superficial layers had been healed. Cytology was falsely positive in one case. The correlation between cytology and clinical course of the disease was extremely satisfactory and cytology must be considered to be a very helpful means of investigation in the follow-up of patients treated by intracavitary irradiation of rectal cancer.

Eleven (5.3%) local failures were observed : two of them were associated with metastatic lymph nodes in the mesorectum. Most local failures (seven) occurred during the first 2 years and may be considered as lack of local control. This demonstrates the usefulness of the assesment of the scar on the first weeks following the irradiation. Four recurrences occurred between the 3rd and the 5th year; no local failure was observed after the 5th year. Three patients were inoperable either because of the extent of the disease in the pelvis or because of their poor general condition. Eight underwent subsequent surgery, either AP resection (seven cases) or anterior resection (one case). Three patients are alive and well, disease-free more than 5 years after operation. One patient died post-operatively; four died from cancer extension. Some illustrative case histories of local failures are given here.

Female aged 63: Polypoid, slightly infiltrating, well-differentiated adenocarcinoma, 3 cm in diameter, located 2 cm above the anal canal, seen in April 1959. Contact X-ray therapy 10 000 R in four applications during period 2–28 April 1959. Radium implant to the base of the tumour on 16th June because of an area of hardening in the rectal wall in the treated area: three needles of 4 mg radium – dose 2 500 rad. Good initial result. Induration considered as local recurrence was mentioned in July 1961, 2 years after treatment. AP resection on 26 August 1961. The operative specimen confirmed adenocarcinoma in the rectal wall. No nodes involved. Patient alive and well in January 1981. She is 85 years old (obs. RON).

Male aged 61: Polypoid, mobile, well-differentiated adenocarcinoma 2.8 cm in diameter located 13 cm above the anal verge, very close to the rectosigmoid junction. Contact X-ray thrapy 13 000 R in four applications from 3 October till 9 November 1961. Irradiation difficult because of the high location of the tumour. Disappearance of the lesion. Five months later, discovery of a malignant polyp situated 1 cm above the primary tumour, too highly located to be irradiated. Abdominoperineal resection on 16 May 1962. No node involved in the operative specimen, which confirmed the presence of a recurrence, very close to the treated area. Patient alive and well in July 1981. He is 80 years old (obs. DUT).

The latter case of local failure was related to the site of the tumour and to the poor accessibility of the lesion close to the rectosigmoid junction.

Male aged 73, in rather poor general health: Protuberant, mobile, fairly well differentiated adenocarcinoma, 2.8 cm in diameter, located 12 cm above the anal verge. The lesion, hard and rather infiltrating was situated astride a valve. Irradiation by contact X-ray therapy: 10 000 R in four applications between 14 April and 9 May 1975. A booster dose of 2 000 rad was delivered to the bed of the tumour by iridium fork in 15 h on 18 June 1975. Apparent primary healing was observed. However, on 21 July 1978, induration of the scar was found at the follow-up endoscopy and considered as a local failure. The patient underwent an anterior resection on 8 September 1978. Pathology confirmed local failure without metastatic nodes. He made a good recovery but died 18 months later on 25 April 1980 from cardiovascular disease, without recurrence of cancer. He was 78 years old (obs. CHA).

Female aged 60: Rather large, ulcerative and proliferating, mobile, well-differentiated adenocarcinoma 5 cm in length, 3 cm in width, located 5–10 cm above the anal verge. Irradiation by contact X-ray therapy: dose 13 000 R in four applications and two overlapping fields for the first two applications, from 29 September till 4 November 1971. A booster dose was given to the bed of the tumour by radium implant on 25 January 1972, using four radium needles 4 cm long, 4 mg radium each for 53 h. Dose delivered 2 200 rad. Good primary result with little fibrotic scar. On 25 July 1972, 6 months after completion of irradiation, a small proliferating lesion, 2 cm in diameter, was discovered at the upper limit of the tumour. A biopsy showed adenocarcinoma. The patient underwent an AP resection on 7 October 1972. The operative specimen confirmed the recurrence at the border at the irradiated site, with superficial infiltration of the rectal wall. No tumour in the centre of the irradiated area. No metastatic nodes. Patient alive and well in October 1981 (obs. ROU) nine years after Surgery (obs. ROU).

The latter is one of the rare cases of marginal recurrence due to the lack of homogeneity of the irradiation. This recurrence could have been controlled by supplementary irradiation using contact and iridium, but the site of the relapse was not easily accessible to palpation. Furthermore, it was thought to be more invasive than it actually was.

In addition to the four patients described above, two further patients underwent radical excision for fibrotic scars wrongly considered to be local failures by a surgeon who disagreed with the views of the radiotherapist responsible for the initial treatment. Both these patients died post-operatively.

Nodal Failures. The digital search for metastatic nodes in the mesorectum should be carried out systematically at every follow-up examination, after local control of low-lying tumours, up to the 5th year, because some metastatic lymph nodes may appear as late as 2–3 years after initial treatment. The radiotherapist should not be content with the assessment of the suppleness and the normal appearance of the area treated by intracavitary irradiation, he must perform a careful digital examination of the rectal and perirectal tissue, especially above the level of the primary tumour. In most patients, a distance of 10 cm above the anal margin can be reached by the index finger. As previously pointed out, the posterior and lateral part of the perirectal structures must be examined with particular care. The discovery of a hard nodule which was not present at the previous examination prompts an immediate surgical approach in order to check its nature.

All patients treated for low-lying tumours at the Centre Léon Bérard underwent during the follow-up period a systematic search for metastatic nodes in the mesorectum and in the lowest part of the pelvis, especially after 1965. In 12 cases (5.8%) indurated metastatic nodules were found either in the mesorectum (ten cases), or along the hypogastric chain against the pelvic wall (two cases). Six patients were inoperable and died. Six had subsequent surgery: four AP resections, two perirectal lymphadenectomies. One patient died post-operatively, two died from cancer; three have been alive and well, disease-free, for more than 5 years. Among these patients cured by surgery are the two who had lymphadenectomy without bowel resection. Both of them are alive without recurrence more than 9 years after surgery. The following are examples of regional node recurrence:

Male aged 57: Proliferating and slightly ulcerative moderately well-differentiated adenocarcinoma, freely mobile, 4 cm in diameter, located at 7 cm above the anal verge.

Irradiation by contact X-ray therapy: dose 11 500 R in four applications from 3 May 1971 till 17 June 1971. Irradiation by two fields for the first two treatments, by one field for the last two applications. Good primary result. Scar extremely supple, with some telangiectases. On 10 November 1972, discovery at the follow-up examination of a hard nodule 2 cm in diameter in the rectal wall, approximately 2 cm above the irradiated area, which appeared normal. The node was located in the same quadrant as the primary tumour.

On 13 December 1972, 18 months after the completion of irradiation, the patient underwent a perirectal lymphadenectomy. The node palpated was easily recongnized; no other hard nodules were felt. The surgeon decided not to perform a radical excision, but only a lymphadenectomy. The node was involved by an adenocarcinoma, with some colloid formation. No other metastatic node in the operative specimen. The patient is alive and well, without any recurrence or any intestinal trouble, in December 1981, more than 9 years after surgery (obs. RON).

Female aged 48: Ulcerative and exophytic well-differentiated adenocarcinoma, located 8 cm above the anal verge. The lesion, 3 cm in diameter, was freely mobile.

Irradiation by contact X-ray therapy: dose 12 500 R in four applications, from 28 June till 27 July 1972. Rapid shrinkage of the tumour and complete disappearance at the end of treatment.

On 9 September 1972, 6 weeks after the last application of contact X-ray therapy, at the first follow-up examination, discovery of a small indurated nodule 1 cm in diameter, approximately 2 cm above the treated area on the same quadrant. The scar was normal.

On 25 October 1972 the patient underwent a perirectal lymphadenectomy. The hard lymph node was easily found. No other hard nodules, no liver metastasis. The surgeon performed only a lymphadenectomy without bowel resection. In the operative speciman, only one node was involved. Rapid recovery. Patient disease-free without any intestinal trouble in December 1981, more than 9 years after conservative surgery (obs. PRO.)

Both these case reports demonstrate the possibility of conservation of the rectum in those very rare cases where the primary tumour has been controlled and involvement of only one lymph node was detected easily by systematic palpation of the rectal wall above the primary lesion on follow-up examination.

In four cases a suspect nodule was found in the perirectal region above the treated area. All these patients underwent surgical exploration either by abdominal, by transanal, or by transperineal approach. Histological examination of the specimens showed that there was no malignant tissue and only fibrotic tissue or cytosteatonecrosis. All these patients have been cured for more than 5 years. One case is reported here:

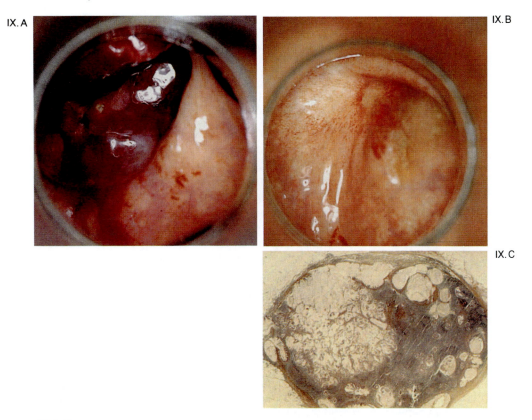

Plate 6

Fig. IX. A. Polypoid adenocarcinoma before treatment.

Fig. IX. B. The same after contact X-ray therapy. Good recovery of the rectal wall. The appearance of the mucosa is almost normal, except for some telangiectasia.

Fig. IX. C. Same patient. Histologic preparation of a metastatic nodule found at follow-up examination one year after contact X-ray therapy. The metastatic lymph node was located in the meso-rectum, 4 cm above the site of the primary tumor. No other node palpated. A lymphadenectomy without bowel resection was performed. Patient alive and well more than nine years later.

Female aged 37: Polypoid, well-differentiated adenocarcinoma 2 cm in diameter, freely mobile, situated 6 cm above the anal verge. Contact X-ray therapy from 18 February till 24 March 1972. Dose 14 000 R in four applications. Normal scar. No residual disease.

Discovery on 21 June 1974, 2 years after treatment, of a hard nodule 1 cm in diameter in the mesorectum, 2 cm above the irradiated area, in the same quadrant as the primary tumour. The patient underwent a laparotomy and a perirectal lymphadenectomy on 9 July 1974. The nodule stuck to the rectal wall was found and removed, as well as lymph nodes. The pathology showed that it was a fibrous node without any malignant tissue. The patient is alive and well in July 1981, 9 years after treatment (obs. CAS).

When the relationship between the number of failures and the size and the configuration of the tumour is examined, the rate of local failures is not statistically higher in tumours bigger than 3 cm (2%) than in smaller tumours (4.6%), whereas the rate of nodal failures is higher in the first group (10.5%) than in the second group. (4%).

In the group of local failures were included two cases with combined local and nodal failures. If one includes these two cases in the group of nodal failures, the rate of nodal failure for ulcerative lesion (14%) is in the same range as the 12.3% described by Morson for lymphatic spread after examination of operative specimens containing ulcerative cancers confined to the rectal wall.

Among the 23 patients who had local or nodal failures, only seven were cured by surgery (less than one in three), and two died post-operatively. These figures confirm that many patients were poor surgical risks and emphasize the importance of careful follow-up by the radiotherapist in charge of treatment of these patients.

During the follow-up period there is uncertainty about the possibility of lymphatic spread after local control of primary tumours located in the middle part of the rectum between 6 cm and 9 cm from the anal verge. The treated area will be entirely normal, but the clinical search for pararectal metastatic lymph nodes cannot be carried out because the rectal wall above the primary tumour is not within reach of the examining finger. In such cases, the possibility of mesenteric and perirectal lymphadenectomy may be considered in good-risk patients under the age of 55. This operation does not have serious complications, and may be performed as a safety measure. Two examples of such a procedure are described here:

Female aged 39: Polypoid, well-differenciated adenocarcinoma 2.5 cm in diameter, located on the posterior wall of the rectum 6 cm above the anal verge. The tumour was astride a valve. Contact X-ray therapy 12 000 R, in four applications, from 25 July till 1 September 1972. The first treatment was applied through two overlapping fields. Normal shrinkage of the tumour, which had disappeared at the end of treatment. Because of the location of the tumour astride a valve, a supplementary treatment by radium implant was performed on 8 November 1972. A booster dose of 2 000 rad was given by three radium needles of 2 mg.

On 10 January 1973, an elective perirectal lymphadenectomy was performed accompanied by a subtotal hysterectomy for uterine myoma. No node involvement. Patient alive and well in December 1981, 9 years after treatment. (obs. GOU)

Male aged 25: Ulcerative and proliferating, freely mobile, well-differentiated adenocarcinoma, 2 cm in diameter, located in the left rectal wall, 7 cm above the anal verge. Contact X-ray therapy, 10 500 R in four applications, between 20 September and 2 November 1977. Shrinkage of the tumour, which was not visible in rectoscopy at the end of treatment. The base of the tumour remained slightly indureated. Iridium implant with two radioactive wires on 14 November 1977, dose 4 500 rad. Dosage of CEA normal.

On 20 January 1978, lymphadenectomy mesenteric and perirectal. No node involved. No liver metastasis. Alive and well, disease-free, in December 1981, more than 4 years after treatment (obs. FOU).

In conclusion, follow-up examination is an integral part of local treatment and makes demands on both the radiotherapist and the patient, who must be aware of the necessity for regular check-up. This follow-up creates a special relationship between doctor and patient and may lead to the need for a subsequent surgical approach with a good prospect of cure or control of any local or lymphatic recurrence.

e) Problem of Rectal Adenocarcinomas of the Juxta-anal Area

Rectal cancers arising in the juxta-anal area must be distinguished from cancers of the lower rectum with spread to the anus, and from synchronous colonic and anal adenocarcinomas. There have been very few publications concerned with primary adenocarcinomas of the anal canal. These tumours are usually included among cancers of the lower third of the rectum and treated by AP resection.

They are situated astride the anorectal junction and always infiltrate the sphincter. This, to a greater or lesser degree, is the reason why they are considered not to be suitable for conservative treatment. In almost all articles devoted to local excision or electrocoagulation, tumours in this position are excluded because conservative surgery would result in disorders of anal function and/or local recurrences. If the lesion is not extensive (4 cm or less) and does not involve more than one-quarter of the anal circumference, the possibility of conservative treatment by irradiation may be considered for high surgical risk patients or those adamant in their refusal of a permanent colostomy.

Rectal adenocarcinomas arising in the juxta-anal area rarely present as polypoid, purely protuberant tumours. From an early stage they are ulcerative and more infiltrating than cancers arising in the mid-rectum, because there is no space for them to grow outwards in the infundibular-shaped juxta-anal area. Sometimes they are exophytic in their rectal part and ulcerative in their anal part. Most of these tumours are located in the anterior half of the anorectal junction. They may look like squamous cell carcinomas of the anal canal, but they tend to narrow the anal orifice less than the true anal cancers do.

In the majority of cases, these lesions are amenable to radical excision. However, in some cases intracavitary irradiation is able to give the patient a chance of cure with preservation of anal function.

It should be borne in mind that, using irradiation, the reaction and the chances of control of the tumour are not the same as those in the case of carcinoma of the rectal ampulla. The underlying sphincter muscle is prone to necrosis and the narrowing of the canal dictates a special approach to this type of lesion. Treatment is based either on a combination of external irradiation by cobalt-60 and iridium implant, or on contact X-ray therapy possibly followed by iridium implant.

The application of contact X-ray therapy in the anal area is not so easy as in the rectal lumen. Local anaesthesia of the anal sphincter is required to relax anal spasm. A special treatment applicator with a visor is needed to prevent the normal rectal mucosa prolapsing into the end of the applicator. Because of the consistency of the sphincter area, the rectal tumour does not present in the front of the applicator, but obliquely into the lumen. Two overlapping fields are commonly used, an upper directed to the rectal part of the tumour, and a lower directed to the anal part. The purpose of contact X-ray therapy is to destroy the exophytic part of the lesion, to reduce its size and to decrease the invaded area.

The treatment consists of three to four applications at 50 kV, 1 mm Al, 2 000 R each, over a period of 8–10 weeks. The free interval between each session is 2–3 weeks. The long overall treatment time is used to protect normal structure and to decrease the risk of necrosis.

One and a half months later, an ulcerative or nodular lesion remains, which may require an iridium implant. This is carried out in the same way as for squamous cell carcinoma of the anal canal (the technique is described in Section B, Chapter XII). The dose delivered varies from 2 000 to 4 000 R according to the thickness of the residual lesion. Usually nor more than four iridium wires are needed.

If the tumour is more infiltrating than exophytic or has a hard consistency, a combined treatment with cobalt-60 and iridium-192 implant may be applied, according to a protocol rather similar to that which is used in the curative treatment of anal canal squamous cell carcinoma. It consists of:

1. Cobalt-60: 3 000 rad at 5 cm depth, by a perineal field 7 × 7 cm in ten fractions over a period of 17 days
2. Iridium-192 implant: booster dose of 2 000 rad carried out 6 weeks later.

The anal area is much more sensitive than the rectal ampulla, and the reaction after irradiation much more severe. Whereas healing is simple and easy after intracavitary irradiation of cancer of the lower half of the rectum, irradiation of cancer of the juxta-anal area may give rise to painful necrotic ulceration, which may make local control difficult to assess because of the hard consistency of underlying sphincteral muscle. Moreover, the digital examination gives rise to pain and spasm, and clinical examination may require general anaesthesia.

Digital, endoscopic, and especially repeated cytological examinations of scrape smears are helpful in distinguishing between necrotic ulcers and failure of local control. These may often be associated.

The chance of cure of limited well-differentiated adenocarcinoma of the anorectal junction is much lower than for cancer of the rectal ampulla, but in elderly or poor-risk patients this method is justifiable with care. Radical surgery can always be performed subsequently if this treatment fails.

Experience at the Centre Léon Bérard. Irradiation of adenocarcinoma located at the anorectal junction can only be considered if three conditions are met:

1. Patients must be poor risk, and the likelihood of death subsequent to AP resection is considered to be especially high.
2. The tumour should be less than 4 cm in diameter and not too deeply infiltrating.
3. Only low-grade malignancy adenocarcinoma can be considered.

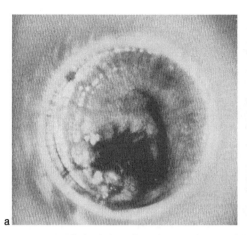 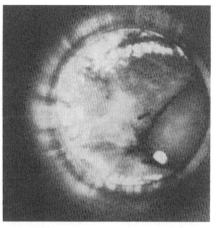

Fig. 16a, b. Limited ulcerative adenocarcinoma of the juxta-anal area in an elderly poor-risk patient. **a** before treatment; **b** after treatment by contact X-ray therapy. Local control of the tumour. Patient died 4 years later from intercurrent disease

Table 13. Statistics regarding treatment of juxta-anal adenocarcinomas measuring less than 4 cm in diameter[a]

Modality	No. of cases
Contact X-ray therapy	8
Contact X-ray therapy + iridium implant	8
Cobalt-60 + iridium implant	23
Iridium implant	5

[a] Centre Léon Bérard.

Forty-four cases were treated at the Centre Léon Bérard between 1965 and 1977; all of them were followed-up over 3 years.

The modality of irradiation varied accordingly to the configuration of the tumour. The distribution of modalities is given in Table 13.

The average age of the patients was 77 years; 19 patients were aged 80 or older. The results are summarized in Table 14. Of the 44 patients treated, 23 (52%) were alive and well, disease-free, for more than 3 years. Among this group of 23 patients, two underwent an AP resection for local failure: 21 have normal anal function. In seven cases painful ulcerative reaction occurred which healed spontaneously in less than 3 months. Ten have been cured for more than 5 years.

Twenty-one patients died – 17 of cancer (38%), five after having had a radical excision. Almost all local failures occurred during the 1st year, and can be considered as primary treatment failure. One patient died of groin metastasis; two died of distant metastasis after local control of the anorectal tumour. One patient died post-operatively; three died of intercurrent disease before 3 years.

The figures given in Table 14 show that careful irradiation applied to patients selected according to their general condition and to the size and configuration of the tumour gives chance of cure in one case in two (Fig. 16a, b).

Table 14. Juxta-anal adenocarcinomas less than 4 cm in diameter: Results of irradiation in poor-risk patients[a]

No. of cases	Alive and well > 3 years	Death		
		Cancer	Interc. disease	Postop.
44	23[b] (52%)	17[c] (38%)	3	1

[a] Centre Léon Bérard
[b] Two after surgery; ten cured at 5 years.
[c] Five after surgery.

It should be remembered that these cases would be suitable for major surgery if they were not in a poor-risk group. Follow-up examination should be particularly careful in the 1st year, so that local failure can be selected at an early stage. In this series only one severe complication (urinary fistula) was seen following salvage surgery.

In conclusion, it may be stated that irradiation has an important role in the management of limited juxta-anal rectal cancer, and can often preserve anal function in patients who are a poor surgical risk.

f) Indications

The indications for intracavitary irradiation are generally the same of those for any local treatment and include the following requirements:
1. The tumour should be well- or moderately well-differentiated adenocarcinoma (the tumour grade is based on multiple biopsies).
2. The tumour should be mobile and readily accessible to the treatment applicator.
3. The tumour should not exceed 5 cm in length and 3 cm in width.
4. There should be no palpable lymph nodes in the mesorectum.
5. The patient must undergo regular long-term follow-up.

Three groups of tumours are to be considered: those with their upper edge palpable but not invading the anus; those located 9–12 cm from the anal verge; and those invading the anal area.

Tumours with Their Upper Edge Palpable but Not Invading the Anus. Most with the upper edge palpable, but not invading the anus, would be suitable for a radical operation with a permanent colostomy if treated by surgery.

Polypoid cancers arising in this area are the most suitable for intracavitary irradiation and are easily controlled by this means whatever their size (under 5 cm) or the age and condition of the patient. Contact X-ray therapy may be combined with an iridium implant if the bed of the tumour appears indurated (Fig. 17).

Limited, mobile, ulcerative cancers can be accepted for this treatment as long as the 3rd-week test demonstrates that the tumour is still confined to the rectal wall. In all such cases, an iridium implant is performed 1 month after completation of contact X-ray therapy. This has proved satisfactory, especially in poor surgical risk patients.

Intracavitary Irradiation of Rectal Tumours

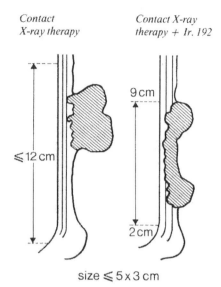

Fig. 17. Polypoid well-differentiated adenocarcinomas smaller than 5 × 3 cm up to 12 cm from the anal verge are suitable for contact X-ray therapy. Ulcerative carcinomas of the lower two-thirds of the rectum are suitable for a conservative treatment by contact X-ray therapy and iridium-192 implant as long as they are confined to the bowel wall (3rd week test); their size must not exceed 5 × 3 cm

Young or middle-aged patients (under 55) are informed of the necessity of an exploratory laparotomy with inferior mesenteric and perirectal lymphadenectomy within the first 3 months following the completion of irradiation.

Tumours Located 9–12 cm from the Anal Verge. Tumours located 9–12 cm from the anal verge are not easily palpated and can usually be treated by a restorative surgical procedure. Intracavitary irradiation is only applicable to localized polypoid rectal cancers less than 3 cm in diameter, because two overlapping fields of contact X-ray therapy are not used at this level.

Limited ulcerative cancers can also be considered, but in such cases intracavitary irradiation is reserved for poor-risk patients and should not be applied to fit patients.

Tumours Invading the Anal Area. When a tumour sits astride the anorectal junction, conservative surgery is excluded. Intracavitary irradiation, combined or not with cobaltherapy, is the only means of preserving the anus and should be applied exclusively to poor surgical risk patients. The technique is different from that which is used for adenocarcinoma of the rectal ampulla, because of the risk of radionecrosis. The chances of control of tumours of the anorectal junction by irradiation are not negligible (23 of 44 cases in the series of patients treated at the Centre Léon Bérard), but this irradiation should be reserved for elderly patients in poor general condition.

VII. Comparison of Surgical and Radiotherapeutic Methods of Local Therapy

The three principal methods of local treatment considered in Chapter V were local excision, electrocoagulation, and intracavitary irradiation. Each aims to achieve complete eradication of the tumour locally with minimal morbidity and preservation of sphincter function. Which is best?
The techniques may be compared according to the following criteria: (a) mode of action, (b) conditions of application, (c) results, and (d) follow-up.

1. Mode of Action

Local excision results in total excision of the tumour, and the specimen is then processed for histological assessment as to its grade of differentiation, the extent of spread through the rectal wall, and the completeness of the removal.

With electrocoagulation and intracavitary irradiation, the tumour is destroyed by heat or by ionizing radiation respectively. The degree of differentiation of the tumour can only be assessed by multiple biopsies performed before treatment is started. Although "total biopsy"' is more accurate than multiple biopsies, the assessment of the grade of malignancy by biopsies, has proved satisfactory in our experience at the Centre Léon Bérard.

When electrocoagulation is used, the surgeon is able to note the appearance and the consistency of the normal tissue during the operation. This indicates the limits of the invaded area. The radiotherapist, too, is able to determine the target volume by the degree of infiltration of each tumour. Contact X-ray therapy is both progressive and selective. The four applications of X-rays are separated by intervals of 1–3 weeks. During this period, the response of the tumour to treatment usually gives a clear idea of its limits. In contrast to electrocoagulation, which destroys all tissues, irradiation has a differential effect related to the degree of radiosensitivity of neoplastic and normal tissues. Careful examination of these changes before each treatment allows the radiotherapist some means of assessing the extent of infiltration.

2. Conditions of Application

Surgical methods require admission to hospital and include a general or caudal anaesthetic. This admission may be anything from a few days to 2–3 weeks. Local excision is a safe technique with minimal morbidity. However, HAWLEY and RITCHIE (1980, St. Mark's Hospital) noted one post-operative death in a patient who had a transsphincteric excision of a large tumour. Early complications are not uncommon after electrocoagulation (24,5% in the series of MADDEN 1979).

Intracavitary contact X-ray therapy is an ambulatory treatment carried out in the out-patient department. It does not require any interruption of the normal activities of patients, which is important psychologically. There is no preparation except for bowel cleansing, and the duration of one application does not exceed 4 min. An intrarectal interstitial iridium implant requires a stay of 3–4 days in hospital. General or caudal anaesthesia is not required, and only local anaesthesia of an area of peri-anal skin to fix a rubber drain is necessary. There is no premedication and no side-effects have been encountered.

Intracavitary irradiation is particularly suitable for elderly patients, for handicapped and mentally confused patients, and those with extremely poor health or on anticoagulating treatment. The only problem is the need for the patient to remain in the knee-chest position for a few minutes.

Contact X-ray therapy is simple and does not require special training. Care must be taken during its application. Each should be done by the same radiotherapist.

3. Control of Tumour

It is generally accepted that tumours larger than 5 cm in diameter should be excluded. Most tumours treated by conservative methods are 4 cm or less in diameter. Pedunculated adenocarcinomas, cancer arising in polyps, and villous tumours are better treated by some form of local excision.

Protuberant, polypoid cancers are, of course, the most suitable tumours for any of the three methods, but electrocoagulation and intracavitary irradiation appear to be safer in some circumstances. When this type of cancer is treated by intracavitary irradiation, the failure rate is especially low (3,8%), whilst a number of failures after local excision have been controlled by irradiation.

Ulcerative cancers are usually associated with significant local spread, and the risk of lymph node involvement is at least twice that for polypoid cancers. Local control is achieved less frequently whatever the modality of treatment. Most ulcerative cancers are more amenable to destruction by electrocoagulation or irradiation than to removal by local excision.

Electrocoagulation can destroy cancers which have spread beyond the rectal wall, whereas the action of intracavitary irradiation (contact X-ray therapy + iridium implant) is limited to the rectal wall. For the radiotherapist, the distinction between the tumours confined to the rectal wall and those that have spread beyond is generally easy. The place of repeated clinical and cytological examinations has been stressed, and gives a clear idea of the end result. As long as the ulcerative cancer is confined to the rectal wall, the chance of local control by intracavitary irradiation is at least equal to and probably exceeds that following electrocoagulation. TURNBULL (1974), who had a long experience with electrocoagulation, was convinced of the advantages of intracavitary irradiation for polypoid and ulcerative tumours confined to the rectal wall, selected by carefully defined criteria.

Ulcerative carcinomas arising in association with villous tumours are best treated by surgery.

One method may have an advantage over another, according to the level of the tumour in the rectum. Electrocoagulation is not advisable for tumours of the upper third of the rectum, because of the risk of perforation into the peritoneal cavity (two cases in the MADDEN 1979 series). Intracavitary irradiation is easily applied to these tumours as long as they are accessible. Local excision is more difficult, and a transsphinteric approach may be necessary. Intracavitary irradiation does, therefore, have certain advantages compared with other techniques for treating polypoid tumours of the upper third of the rectum.

The site of the tumour on the anterior, posterior, or lateral wall of the rectum is important, since each presents difficulties of a particular kind.

For instance, tumours of the anterior wall of the rectum in female patients are often considered unsuitable for electrocoagulation because of the risk of rectovaginal fistula. After intracavitary irradiation, even if an iridium implant is used, there should be no danger of fistula formation of the technique is carefully applied. At the Centre Léon Bérard only one rectovaginal fistula has been documented. This occurred in 1961 in a patient 77 years old. This fistula followed excessive irradiation of a large ulcerative adenocarcinoma during curietherapy with radium needles. It required a temporary colostomy which was closed 3 months later after the fistula had healed spontaneously. This patient died 12 years later, free from cancer. No other rectovaginal fistulas have been observed since 1961, although more ulcerative tumours have been treated during the past 2 decades.

Conversely, some cancers of the lowest part of the posterior wall of the rectum, located in the concavity of the sacral bone, may be difficult to irradiate because of poor accessibility by the treatment applicator. Electrocoagulation or local excision by the transsphincteric approach are probably more suitable for such cases.

One of the main advantages of intracavitary irradiation is its application to limited adenocarcinomas at the anorectal junction. These tumours invade or encroach on the sphincter and are considered unsuitable for local excision or electrocoagulation because of the danger of incontinence or local failure. Irradiation is difficult, but control of limited adenocarcinomas can be achieved in poor-risk patients, with preservation of anal function. This is possible because of the progressive selectivity of irradiation. X-ray doses are closely adapted to the target volume, and the irradiated area is limited to prevent severe radionecrosis with damage to the sphincter.

4. Follow-up

The aim of follow-up is early detection of local and nodal failure, after primary local control has been achieved. Local failures always produce induration and a change in the consistency of the treated area, which may be associated with polypoid or ulcerative changes. The detection of these changes is easy if the scar is supple or slightly fibrotic without stricture, as is the case after intracavitary irradiation or local excision. The development of a hard nodule can be more difficult to assess after electrocoagulation, since the scar is harder and retracted, with a certain degree of stricture formation. If the original tumour was situated low in the rectum, the detection of a metastatic lymph node above this site requires careful digital examination, and this is only possible if there is no narrowing of the treated area. Such examination may be impossible following electrocoagulation, because of the retracted scar.

5. Conclusion

In conclusion, intracavitary irradiation is able to control all tumours suitable for local excision as safely and more simply than other methods of local treatment. The combination of contact therapy with iridium implant competes favourably with electrocoagulation with the exception of: (a) deeply infiltrating tumours, which should not be treated by local treatment anyway; and (b) those rare tumours found on the posterior wall of the rectum in the sacral concavity.

VIII. Intracavitary Irradiation as a Supplementary Procedure After Local Excision – Problem of Villous Adenomas

GOLIGHER (1977) has emphasized the "difficult problem that confronts a surgeon, when an apparently benign adenoma or villous papilloma has been removed by local excision or diathermy snare and the pathologist reports that the lesion is in fact an invasive carcinoma". Published series show that local and nodal recurrences may occur not infrequently, especially during the first 2 years following excision. The first principle is to check the grade of malignancy of the tumour. If it is high-grade (poorly differentiated or colloid carcinoma), the only reliable procedure is a radical excision, which should be performed without delay (LOCKHART-MUMMERY and DUKES 1952). Secondly, it is important to ensure that the local excision has been complete. In a series of local excisions for rectal adenocarcinoma published by HAWLEY and RITCHIE (1980) at St. Mark's Hospital, of 42 patients six underwent an early reoperation, either because of the grade of malignancy of the carcinoma or because the excision was considered inadequate. Of the 36 remaining, seven (20%) developed local recurrences and underwent a radical excision; three (8%) had nodal involvement in the operative specimen. Two patients (5,5%) died of cancer. The follow-up was between 1 and 30 years.

If the tumour is of average-grade malignancy, extending deeply into the submucosa, there are three options:
1. Careful follow-up
2. A radical excision to control the bed of the tumour and remove the lymph nodes, which may be involved in 6%–10% of cases
3. A supplementary conservative procedure such as electrocoagulation or intracavitary irradiation.

If the patient is a poor surgical risk, obese, or with cardiovascular or bronchopulmonary problems, a radical operation might be associated with greater risks than those from lymphatic dissemination. GOLIGHER (1977) has stressed that "under these circumstances, it may be preferable to accept the calculated risk of a conservative procedure above all, if the location of the tumor in the lower rectum implied the sacrifice of the sphincter apparatus, with permanent colostomy", and allows the search of metastatic lymph nodes in the mesorectum by digital examination.

The purpose of supplementary conservative treatment is to lessen the risk of local recurrence. Intracavitary irradiation has proved to be easy to apply to the scar of local excision, by contact X-ray therapy and/or iridium implant. When the scar is flat and easily accessible, contact X-ray therapy 50 kV, 1 mm Al, is performed 1 month after surgery, in three applications separated by a 2-week interval. The dose per treatment is 2000 R, the overall dose of 6000 R being delivered over 4 weeks. It is advisable not to exceed this dose because of the risk of radionecrosis in the area operated on. If the scar is not flat, but fibrotic and irregular, the dose delivered by contact X-ray therapy would not be homogeneous. In such cases, a combination of contact X-ray therapy (two fractions of 2000 R) and an iridium implant delivering 3000–4000 rad is the best approach.

1. Experience at the Centre Léon Bérard

Between 1962 and 1977, 77 patients were irradiated as a prophylactic treatment after local excision of a malignant polyp or a villous papilloma with invasive adenocarcinoma. All the tumours were non-pedunculated, well- or fairly well differentiated adenocarcinomas. Six local failures (7,7%) and one nodal failure were observed; four patients died of cancer, three are alive and well after AP resection. Eleven patients died of intercurrent disease (eight) or second primary cancer (three); 62 (80,5%) patients are alive and well after 3–18 years, 59 with normal anal function and three with colostomy (Table 15).

Table 15. Intracavitary irradiation after local excision for malignant polyp or degenerated villous papilloma[a]

No. of cases	Alive and well > 3 years	Death	
		Cancer	Intercurrent disease
77	62[b] (80,5%)	4 (5,5%)	11 (14,3%)

[a] Centre Léon Bérard.
[b] Three after salvage surgery, 59 with normal anal function.

When one compares the rate of failures observed after intracavitary irradiation following local excision with that of the series of local excision alone of St. Mark's Hospital, it can be seen that irradiation decreases the risk of recurrence after local surgery. Very simple and without any danger, this procedure deserves consideration as a safety measure after local excision, when there is no indication for radical surgery.

Villous adenomas of the rectum are treated surgically. However, intracavitary irradiation must be considered as a first approach or for recurrences in inoperable or poor-risk patients. Villous adenomas with or without signs of degeneration treated by contact X-ray therapy show the same radiation response as rectal adenocarcinomas (RAYMOND et al. 1977).

From a series of 70 cases followed up for more than 5 years one can state that limited villous adenomas can be controlled by contact X-ray therapy, and that the method represents in such cases an alternative to surgery.

Section B
Epidermoid Carcinoma of the Anus

Topographical Distribution of Anal Cancers

It is customary to divide squamous cell cancers of the anus into two groups according to their site of origin: carcinoma of the anal canal, and carcinoma of the anal margin. Unfortunately there is no agreement on the extent of these regions. The Mayo Clinic considers the anal canal to end at the anal verge where the modified skin of the anal canal joins the hair-bearing perineal skin. At St. Mark's Hospital, London, the distal end of the anal canal is taken as the mucocutaneous junction where the dentate line is situated. This variation in the interpretation of anatomical terms makes the comparison of data from different institutions very difficult. Tumours located below the dentate line may be considered as arising from either the anal canal or the anal margin.

In this monograph, the principles described by BEAHRS of the Mayo Clinic (1979) have been adopted, and all tumours arising above the anal verge are considered to be anal canal tumours. Carcinomas arising from the perianal area outside the anal verge, in the region defined by a circle 6 cm in diameter with the anal orifice as the centre, are regarded as carcinomas of the anal margin. This classification [which is apparently accepted by PARKS (1981) from St. Mark's Hospital] has the advantage of correlating with the arrangement of the lymphatics in this area in addition to the clinical data. It will be shown that some tumours arising below the dentate line may give rise to pelvic nodes (see p. 166). The clinician can easily distinguish between tumours of the anal canal and the anal margin, whereas he is often unable to assess accurately whether a lesion encroaches on the dentate line. Moreover, when MORSON (1960) examined operative specimens at St. Mark's Hospital, he found that 10% of cases were unclassified because it was difficult to determine whether the tumours arose above or below the dentate line.

IX. Epidermoid Carcinoma of the Anal Canal

1. Introduction

There have been very few scientific reports on epidermoid carcinoma of the anal canal until recently. This type of tumour has been overshadowed by rectal cancer and considered as a poor relation amongst tumours of the distal part of the bowel, because of its relative rarity. In many institutions, cancers of the anal canal and those of the lower rectum were treated by the same procedure, namely abdominoperineal (AP) resection. Inoperable or unresectable tumours were referred to the radiotherapist for palliative treatment only. At present there is an increasing interest in the study of anal canal carcinoma, and a greater awareness of its different behavior as compared with rectal cancer.

Epidermoid carcinoma of the anal canal is a very peculiar disease. Always palpable and at times visible, it should be easily controlled by radical excision. However, BACON (1964) considered that "if compared with rectal carcinoma, which is less easily diagnosed, anal cancer has a less favorable prognosis and is unpredictable refractory to the therapeutic efforts of medical science". Radical surgery for this type of tumour is less successful than for rectal cancer.

The true nature of epidermoid carcinoma of the anal canal has often not been well understood. There are great differences between squamous cell carcinoma of the anal canal and adenocarcionma of the rectum in the site of involvement, incidence of lymphatic spread, rate of distant metastases, and above all response to radiation therapy.

The therapeutic approach to squamous cell carcinoma of the anal canal should be different from that to rectal adenocarcinoma. A turning-point in treatment has been reached because of the progress made in the use of irradiation initiated in France, and in several American institutions such as the Memorial Sloan Kettering Institute Cancer Centre, New York in 1974 (NEWMANN and QUAN 1976). At St. Mark's Hospital and the Mayo Clinic, squamous cell carcinomas of the anal canal are usually treated by surgery with a permanent colostomy, whereas at the Memorial Hospital this tumour is first treated by a combined approach based on irradiation and chemotherapy, followed a few weeks later by an excision, either radical or local. In Lyon radiation therapy has become the primary management of all carcinomas of the anal canal. It may well be possible to cure more patients with this regimen and at the same time spare many of them a permanent colostomy.

2. Anatomical and Pathological Background

The anal canal begins where the lower end of the rectal ampulla suddenly narrows, and ends at the anal margin. It is a short passage, 3–5 cm long, completely collapsed because of the tonic contraction of the anal sphincters in normal subjects. Embryologically, the anal canal is derived from the ectoderm, whereas the rectum is derived from the endoderm. These origins explain the different cellular types of epithelium and the variation in the response to irradiation of carcinomas arising from anal mucosa and from rectal mucosa.

The anal canal is usually divided into two parts: the upper mucosal part and the lower cutaneous part, the junction of the two being marked by the line of the anal valves about 2 cm from the anal orifice, opposite the middle of the internal sphincter. This level is called the "dentate" or "pectinate" line. Below the dentate line, the anal canal is covered with a modified skin devoid of hair and sebaceous and sweat glands, and closely adherent to the underlying sphincter muscles. At the junction between the anal canal and anal margin there is a gradual transition from columnar, then stratified, epithelium to true skin.

The area between the dentate line and the rectal ampulla consists of a zone less than 2 cm long, which is called the "transitional" or "junctional" zone studied by GRINVALSKY and HELWIG (1956). MORSON (1960) has stressed that the structure of the epithelium in this area is:

"a compromise between the glandular rectal mucosa above and the squamous mucous membrane or modified skin below the level of the valves. The transitional zone is an area of considerable epithelial instability which contains a number of different varieties of epithelium. One can see a transitional type of mucosa resembling urinary tract epithelium, stratified columnar epithelium, and squamous mucous membrane as well as mixed epithelium which may show features of all these varieties and also contains scattered droplets of mucous secretion".

It is not surprising, therefore, that anal canal carcinomas have variable histology (Fig. 18). Most of them are the ordinary squamous type. Typical prickle cell carcinomas which produce much keratin are rare, and many show little evidence of keratinization.

Muco-epidermoid carcinomas may be found in the anal canal. They are very rare. No such case has been observed in the series of the Centre Léon Bérard. This tumour is a type of squamous cell carcinoma which produces mucus as well as keratin (MORSON 1960). Above the dentate line, carcinomas arising from the transitional zone are called transitional carcinomas because they resemble bladder carcinomas. Poorly differentiated tumours may be similar to basal cell carcinomas of the skin and are called "basaloid carcinomas".

In the American literature, all these tumours are called "cloacogenic carcinomas", but the use of this term varies with different authors. Cloacogenic carcinomas represented 50% of anal canal cancers in a report by KLOTZ et al. (1967), but only 20% in a study of the ultrastructure of this type of tumour by GILLESPIE and MACKAY (1978) who identified three types of cloacogenic carcinomas: (a) the well-differentiated cloagenic carcinomas, which resemble urothelial tumours; (b) the poorly differentiated cloacogenic carcinomas, which include basaloid carcinomas; and (c) the pleomorphic carcinomas, which are intermediate forms of transitional carcinomas.

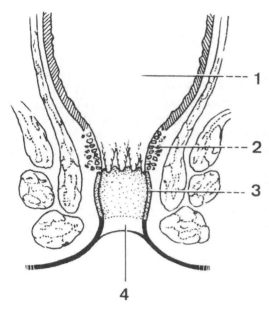

Fig. 18. Different types of carcinoma according to anorectal structures: *1*, rectal mucosa – adenocarcinoma; *2*, upper part of the anal canal, transitional zone – squamous cell carcinoma and cloacogenic, basaloid carcinoma; *3*, lower part of the anal canal, below the dentate line – squamous cell carcinoma; *4*, skin of the external margin of the anus or peri-anal region – squamous cell carcinoma, basal cell carcinoma, Bowen's disease, Paget's disease. NB Colloid carcinoma may arise from the anal ducts situated above the anal valves

BEAHRS and WILSON (1976) included all tumours described as cloacogenic, basaloid, or transitional carcinoma under the heading of basaloid.

MORSON and SOBIN (1964), in their histological classification of intestinal tumours, identified three forms of epidermoid carcinoma of the anal canal: (a) squamous cell carcinoma, resembling squamous carcinoma of the uterine cervix; (b) basaloid carcinoma; and (c) muco-epidermoid carcinoma.

There are a number of simple practical concepts which should be stressed:
1. An accurate picture of the histological type should be obtained by taking multiple biopsies from different areas of the tumour. It is not essential to examine the whole tumour if this practice is followed.
2. Tumours containing different types of epidermoid cells (squamous, basaloid, basisquamous) should be classified as epidermoid.
3. Although the varieties of tumours are interesting from the pathological point of view, it is so far not possible to draw from the histological type of tumour clear indications applicable to the therapeutic approach, and especially to the respective roles of surgery and radiation therapy. STEARNS and QUAN (1970) admit that "these lesions are best considered simply as variants of epidermoid carcinoma, their treatment being based on clinical characteristics and location of the tumors rather than on the cell type". However, an exception should be made for the rare muco-epidermoid carcionomas, which do not respond to radiotherapy as well as the other forms.
4. Most epidermoid carcinomas of the anal canal are poorly differentiated with little keratinization, and considered according to Broders criteria as "highly malignant". This concept does not fit in with our clinical experience, because these tumours in general grow slowly and are often cured by appropriate treatment. Histological features do not seriously influence the prognosis (MORSON

and PANG 1968), except that the more poorly differentiated lesions tend to be diagnosed at a more advanced stage (CORMAN and HAGGITT 1977) and with higher probability of lymphatic spread. (LOYGUE et al. 1981)

Two types of adenocarcinoma arising from the anal canal have been excluded from this study:

1. Adenocarcinoma of the rectal type. Their structure is similar to that of adenocarcinoma of the large bowel and should be included with cancers of the lowest part of the rectum.
2. Colloid carcinoma within anorectal fistula. A special mention must be made of the anal crypts or sinuses of MORGAGNI, which are little pockets situated above the anal valves. These are of some pathological significance because the anal glands or ducts open directly into the apex of an anal crypt. These ducts, which are blind outgrowths of anal crypts, were described by HERMANN and DESFOSSES in 1880. Rarely, colloid carcinomas may arise from the anal ducts. They grow extremely slowly and involve the peri-anal area as well as the perineal soft tissues and skin, and may present as malignant fistulas.

X. General Features

1. Frequency and Sex Distribution

Epidermoid carcinoma of the anal canal is considered to be a rare disease, since it represents 3%–5% of cancers of the large bowel. In fact it is not so rare as it is thought to be, since it represents 12%–15% of the malignant tumours arising in the distal 10 cm of the bowel. In all series there is a predominance of female patients, in contrast to cancers of the rectum and peri-anal area, which are more common in men. The sex ratio in favour of women varies substantially: 3:2, DUKES (1960) and QUAN et al. (1978); 3:1, BEAHRS (1979), BEAHRS and WILSON (1976); 4:1 LOYGUE et al. (1981); 4:1. PILLERON (1973), PILLERON et al. (1970); 5:1, KEY and WHITEHEAD (1980), ESCHWEGE et al. (1979) and for the series from the Centre Léon Bérard. KLOTZ et al. (1967) reported 67% women in a series of 373 cases of cloacogenic carcinoma. No satisfactory explanation has been offered for this sex predilection, and it must be emphasized that anal canal carcinoma is the only one with such female predominance among the epidermoid carcinomas observed in both sexes.

2. Age

The mean age of presentation with anal canal cancer is about 60, with a wide range from the age of 25 to very elderly patients. In contrast to cancer of the rectum, presentation at a young age does not imply a bad prognosis, and carcinomas in this group are not less differentiated than those in older patients. A large number of patients (30%) are poor risks because of their age or other medical problems not related to their cancer.

3. Site

Approximately 40% of tumours are situated above the dentate line, 25% below, and 35% astride it. All tumours involving the dentate line are classified by BEAHRS (1979) and BEAHRS and WILSON (1976) as "anorectal", whereas those in-side the anal canal or on the anal verge but encroaching on the dentate line are classified as "anal canal lesions". Epidermoid carcinoma may occasionally be found in the lower rectum without a direct connection to the anal canal. The presence of these aberrant cancers may be explained by cell metaplasia, or as arising from embryonal rests. They are included in the framework of epidermoid carcinomas of the anal canal and treated along the same lines, although with adaptations to their ectopic location.

4. Configuration

Carcinoma of the anal canal may present a variety of clinical appearances. A very early cancer may resemble a button with nodular elevation of the mucosa, or a warty growth. It may assume one of a number of different appearances and be confused with an anal fissure or thrombosed haemorrhoid, but usually the edge of the lesion feels harder than would normally be expected. Induration is the cardinal sign, but it may sometimes be difficult to assess when there is inflammation or an associated benign lesion such as fistula or haemorrhoids. In these instances the initial diagnosis is often wrong, and only a biopsy will demonstrate malignancy.

Anal canal carcinoma presents as an exophytic, cauliflower-shaped, projecting lesion with limited infiltration of the underlying tissues in fewer than 20% of cases. More commonly it forms either an ulcer with raised everted edges and an indurated base (40%), or a very hard nodular infiltrating mass involving the surrounding structures (40%). The appearance of this particular form of anal cancer, which is easily felt on palpation, must be stressed. The lesion does not project into the anal canal and is covered with swollen mucosa, with little ulceration (Fig. 19). The ulcer is minute compared with the size of the tumour, and the infiltrating submucous part predominates. This presentation is not found with adenocarcinoma of the rectum involving the anal region, and it is usually easy to identify squamous cell carcinomas of the anal canal and adenocarcinomas of the anorectal junction by their appearance. When there is doubt about the diagnosis a generous biopsy must be taken under local or, preferably, general anaesthesia. Otherwise a diagnosis of an inflammatory reaction can be made and the patient may be discharged only to return later with a large and usually inoperable lesion with little hope of cure. At a late stage the growth becomes firmly fixed to the deeper structures projecting and ulcerating in the anal canal and at times completely surrounding the anus.

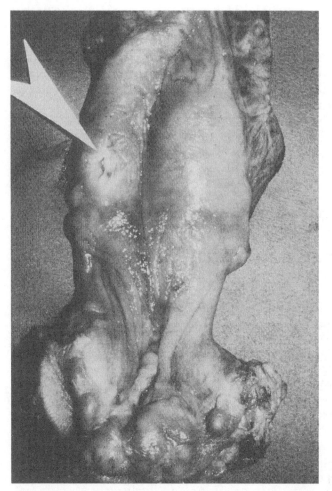

Fig. 19. Operative specimen from AP resection for large squamous cell carcinoma infiltrating more than two-thirds of the circumference of the anal canal, involving the lower part of the rectum. Notice the limited ulceration compared with the bulk of the tumour made up of infiltrating nodules. A pararectal metastatic lymph node found at the rectal digital exmaination is shown by the *white arrow*

5. Tumour Spread

There are three modes of spread: local, regional, and distant.

a) Local Spread

The sphincter is invaded early, because the anal mucosa is bound tightly to underlying muscles. The spread of the growth tends to be annular, producing induration and narrowing of the anal canal. The tumour may extend upwards to the rectal mucosa for a few centimetres, or downwards to the external margin of the anus, and produce ulcer with raised edges in the quadrants involved by the anal canal lesion. The involvement of the anal margin is rarely extensive and in no case does it exceed the volume of the tumour in the anal canal. It is not difficult to distinguish between anal canal cancer spreading downwards to the anal margin and peri-anal cancers with spread upwards into the anal canal.

Posterior tumours may spread directly to the fibrous, fatty, and muscular tissue connecting the anal canal with the coccyx and laterally with the ischiorectal fossa on either side. Anteriorly, in the female, the lowest part of the rectovaginal wall and the perineal body are frequently invaded. The vaginal mucosa remain swollen with intact mucosa for a long time, and the mucosa become ulcerated in late cases only. Downward spread usually involves the deep structures of the perineum, whereas the skin and subcutaneous tissue between anus and vulva remain intact, because of the resistance provided by the arrangement of the anal musculature. In the male the tumour may extend to the bulb of the urethra and the prostate.

b) Regional Spread

There are two routes of regional spread: lymphatic and venous.

Lymphatic spread is more important, because anal canal carcinoma may involve the inguinal as well as the pelvic lymph nodes, irrespective of the size of the tumour and its site below or above the dentate line. Detection of a small tumour does not exclude the risk of lymphatic metastases. The only tumour which one can feel confident has not metastasized is the intramucosal, in situ lesion, which is rarely discovered except in haemorrhoidectomy specimens. The lymphatic networks of the anal canal drain to three groups of nodes: inguinal, pelvic visceral and pelvic parietal.

Inguinal Route. The lower plexuses drain through a series of collecting vessels in the subcutaneous tissue of the genitocrural fold to the inguinal nodes, and especially those in the medial part of the groin. Efferents from these nodes are tributaries of the pelvic group of lymph nodes, successively the retrocrural nodes, which are a direct continuation of the inguinal nodes: the external iliac nodes; and the common iliac nodes. Metastasis to an inguinal node has always been emphasized as one of the most frequent paths of spread in carcinoma of the anus. Involvement of the inguinal nodes is common; it is found in 15%–30% of cases (Table 16). It is always ipsilateral or bilateral, never contralateral. Usually one or a few nodes are involved. Diffuse involvement of all inguinal nodes is rare. Sometimes invasion of the groin is accompanied by a series of satellite nodules of permeation along the skin of the genitocrural area. The prognosis is very poor in this situation. Metastatic inguinal nodes are more common with large tumours than with limited cancers, and more frequent when the tumour is found in the lower part of the anal canal than when it is situated higher up above the dentate line. They occur whatever the configuration of the tumour.

Table 16. Frequency of involvement of inguinal nodes

Author	No. of cases	Rate
SAWYERS (1972)	26	21%
KLOTZ (1967)	373	20%
STEARNS and QUAN (1970)	109	40%
MCCONNELL (1970)	96	25%
BACON (1964)	102	20%
LOYGUE et al. (1981)	149	16%
BEAHRS and WILSON (1976)	146	9%
HAWLEY (personal communication)	195	32,3%
DILLARD et al. (1963)	78	14%
KUEHN et al. (1968)	200	20%

Prognosis of Inguinal Spread. There is a general agreement that the development of metastatic nodes in the groin has a grave prognostic significance and that few patients with inguinal metastasis survive for 5 years. In oncology, whatever the site of the tumour, the involvement of regional lymph nodes decreases significantly the chance of long-term survival, and anal canal cancer conforms to this general rule. However, the prognosis of inguinal metastatic nodes is also related to other factors, such as time of their appearance, extent of the lymphatic spread, stage of the disease, modalities of treatment, and condition of the patient.

Time of Appearance. All authors have noticed that the prognosis differs according to the time of discovery of the metastatic nodes. Prognosis is poor when the inguinal nodes are involved at the patient's first examination. That would mean that the anal tumour was extensive and/or of high malignancy, whereas inguinal metastases appearing subsequently after control of the primary tumour have a better outlook. When metastatic inguinal adenopathy was present at the time of decision before treatment of the anal tumour, GRINNELL (1954), JUDD and DE TAR (1955), and BOND (1960) reported depressing results with no 5-year survivors among the patients treated by AP resection and groin block dissection. At St. Mark's Hosptial, Wolfe (1968) found that 49 of 170 patients had an inguinal involvement when first seen, but only 19 (38,7%) were deemed suitable for block dissection; five (10,2%) of these were alive and well 5 years later, and four had survived 10 years later. STEARNS and QUAN (1970) reported two survivors (14,2%) among 14 patients with simultaneous inguinal metastasis and untreated anal carcinoma.

Subsequent development of inguinal metastasis has a less unfavourable prognostic significance. DILLARD et al. (1963) found that in most patients whose inguinal glands were originally considered to be clinically normal, groin metastases developed within 6 months after treatment of the primary tumour, suggesting that local control of the anal lesion appeared to encourage the development of lymphatic spread. However, some inguinal metastases may occur later, during the first 2 years and even 4, 5, or 6 years after control of the anal lesion. WOLFE (1968) reported 17 patients who developed late groin metatases and were submitted to block dissection; nine (52,9%) were alive and well 5 years later. STEARNS and QUAN (1970) found that 15 (75%) of 20 such patients survived 5 years after groin dissection. GOLDEN and HORSLEY (1976) reviewed the literature and found a 20% 5-year survival rate after groin dissection for synchronous inguinal metastases, versus 59% for metachronous inguinal metastases.

Other Factors. The definitive treatment of metastatic nodes by the most efficient procedure, for instance, block dissection with additive irradiation, is justified for T1, T2 and T3 anal canal cancers. With advanced unresectable anal cancer which has spread to the inguinal lymph nodes, groin block dissection may be considered in each individual case, bearing in mind the chance of local control of the disease by radiation therapy. All these factors interfere with the general condition of the patient. In very elderly or senile patients block dissection is only rarely indicated, whereas a limited removal of two or three involved nodes with additional irradiation can be very helpful.

In the majority of cases inguinal spread can be controlled, and treatment failures are related to local or pelvic spread rather than to groin metastases. However, in some cases the degree of extent of inguinal involvement is so important (unresectable mass, more than 5 nodes involved, association with iliac metastasis) that the cause of death may be directly related to the groin metastasis. This is the case when inguinal adenopathy is associated with haemorrhoidal gland involvement. The chances of control of the disease are very poor, and WOLFE (1968) admitted that palliation is all that can be offered by surgery. It is now recognized that in such cases high doses of radiation therapy applied with a well-planned protocol may give the patient some chance of long-term survival.

Two Pelvic Routes. The *visceral route* follows the distribution of the superior heamorrhoidal vessels upwards to the inferior mesenteric vessels. The collecting lymphatic channels follow the arterial branches along the rectal wall. Their course is interrupted by groups of pararectal nodes. The first of these pararectal nodes are siuated low down, a few centimetres above the junction of the anus and the rectum, along the lateral or posterior wall rather than the anterior wall, which is usually free of nodes. GRINNEL (1954) has noted that the node metastases are usually grouped closer to the primary tumour and found less often at higher levels than in carcinoma of the rectum. Stress must be placed on this point with regard to the possibility of palpation of these nodes. Higher up, the lymphatic channels drain into the nodes situated at the bifurcation of the superior haemorrhoidal artery (Fig. 19).

The *parietal route* is made up of channels which follow the middle haemorrhoid vessels and drain first into the internal iliac group and then into the common iliac group. Some channels run in the hollow of the sacrum to nodes in the presacral area. Efferent channels are tributaries of the aortic lymph nodes, and may extend to the left supraclavicular lymph nodes.

The pelvic lymphatic chains are involved in 10%–46% of patients (Table 17). These figures are drawn from series where patients were treated by radical surgery. They do not give an exact idea of the true rate of metastases, because in most series a certain number of patients have been treated by conservative or palliative procedures. The rate of involvement of pelvic lymph nodes would seem to be between 25% and 35%, although there is wide variation in the incidences reported.

Table 17. Incidence of pelvic metastatic nodes

Author	No. of cases	Rate
GRINNELL (1954)	7/25	28%
DARGENT (1958)	3/30	10%
SEDWICK and WAINSTEIN (1959)	3/28	10,7%
RICHARDS et al. (1962)	14/41	34%
DILLARD et al. (1963)	18/40	45%
BROWN and McKENZIE (1963)	7/19	37%
SAWYERS et al. (1963)	8/42	19%
KLOTZ et al. (1967)	75/378	20%
KUEHN et al. (1968)	45/200	22,5%
HARDCASTLE and BUSSEY (1968)	55/123	44,7%
HARDY et al. (1969)	19/41	46%
MOLLER (1970)	3/16	18,7%
STEARNS and QUAN (1970)	16/67	24%
GOLDEN and HORSLEY (1976)	6/26	23%

In the series of 88 AP resections reported by LOYGUE et al. in 1981, the probability of pelvic lymph node metastasis is related to histological grading (range from 9% to 47%) and to the size of the tumour (25% for tumours sized not more than 4 cm, 50% for tumours larger than 4 cm).

Involvement of pelvic lymph nodes is usually found when the tumour is large and infiltrating, but it may be seen in small early lesions of the anal canal. MORSON (1960) felt that heamorrhoidal gland involvement is extremely rare in cancers located below the dentate line, if it ever occurs, and that this observation justifies the current practice of local excision of these tumours where possible. In fact, *involvement of the pelvic nodes may occur in those patients with carcinoma of the lower part of the anal canal even at an early stage.* SAWYERS (1972) mentioned one patient with perirectal lymph node involvement out of 16 patients with tumour of the lower anal canal. KLOTZ et al. (1961) noticed 15% of perirectal nodal metastasis in 166 cancers situated below the dentate line. Three such cases observed at the Centre Léon Bérard are reported on pp. 166, 167. This pattern of lymphatic spread emphasizes the necessity of including the tumours located below the dentate line as well as tumours situated in the upper part of the anal canal under the heading of carcinoma of the anal canal.

Venous Spread. The tumour may penetrate the walls of veins and then poliferate intravascularly, producing a thickening of the wall. Some in-transit metastases may give rise to hard nodules of permeation consisting of clusters of cells growing around the periphery of the vascular pedicle. These nodules may resemble metastatic lymph nodes on gross examination, but microscopic examination shows that they do not contain any lymphatic structures and are centred on a vascular pedicle (Fig. 29).

c) Distant Spread

Haematogenous spread is not so common in anal canal cancer as in cancer of the rectum. Distant metastases to the liver or lung occur in fewer than 10% of cases. KUEHN et al. (1968) in a series of 200 cases collected from 31 hospitals in Connecticut, reported 13 liver metastases and six lung metastases, usually bilateral. They are almost exclusively observed in advanced tumours which have invaded the anorectal junction.

6. Symptoms and Diagnosis

In the early stages, patients with anal canal cancer are often symptom-free or do not have sufficient symptoms to seek medical advice. Limited tumours are only discovered at routine examination for what is called "haemorrhoids". This is why the disease is discovered late in more than 60% of patients.

Contrary to what is often described, pain is not an early symptom of cancer of the anal canal. For a long period of time, pain is absent. When it occurs, it is located in the anal area with radiation to the perineum, the sacrum, and the buttocks. When an anal carcinoma bleeds, the loss is usually very slight, with a small red mark on the paper during cleansing (BENSAUDE and NORA 1968). The patient may also complain of discomfort or itching around the anus. These signs are often followed by a symptom-free period of 2–3 months, and subsequent onset of symptoms of a similar nature may not alarm the patient. The beginning of the disease is so imprecise that the duration of the symptoms before diagnosis is difficult to assess in most cases.

In other cases, a lump may be felt in the anus or in the posterior part of the vagina. Some patients present with disturbances of bowel habit wrongly attributed to constipation, or with pain on defecation. Incontinence due to malignant infiltration of the sphincters and the symptoms of a rectovaginal fistula are only encountered in very advanced cases.

The problem of diagnosis is well summarized by QUAN (1978), who stressed that

symptoms produced by anal canal neoplasm are not different from those seen with more common inflammatory and non-malignant conditions, and are usually non-specific. A patient with either condition may describe bleeding, pain, burning, pruritus, discomfort, drainage, sensation of a mass and so on. These common complaints, if considered trivial on the part of the patient and physician may delay an early diagnosis of a malignant tumor in the anal region.

In many series, several patients were treated for haemorrhoids or for anal fissure before the diagnosis of carcinoma was made. GOLIGHER (1975) emphasized that induration is the feature that should raise the suspicion of carcinoma, even with the most atypical lesion. Sometimes, an inguinal metastatic node may be the first sign of an unsuspected and symptom-free anal canal cancer. An isolated node can be mistaken for a hernia or an inflammatory node, and the error in diagnosis may cause serious delay in treatment. Needle or open biopsy will demonstrate the true nature of the node, and lead to proper examination of the anal canal and lower rectum. In three cases observed at the Centre Léon Bérard, inguinal metastatic adenopathy occurred 6–12 months before the discovery of the anal canal cancer.

The case reported below illustrates the sort of error in diagnosis which may be fatal.

Female aged 67. Lung tuberculosis treated 38 years earlier. Right inguinal adenopathy considered possibly related to the tuberculosis and treated medically for 3 months. Then an excision of the node showed that it was a lymph node involved by squamous cell carcinoma. Clinical evaluation was performed, except for rectal digital examination. The patient was seen 7 months later, a few days after a rectal bleeding which was the only symptom of the anal lesion.

Clinical examination showed: (a) a huge infiltrating squamous cell carcinoma of the anterior part of the anal canal involving the lower part of the rectum and of the rectovaginal wall; (b) a big external iliac lymph node 6 cm in diameter, fixed to the right pelvic structures; (c) a metastatic lymph node 3 cm in diameter in the genitocrural fold. Pyelography showed a displacement of the right pelvic ureter related to the pelvic mass. Lymphangiography demonstrated a large defect in the right pelvic lymphatic chain.

The patient underwent palliative irradiation with complete remission for 2 years, and died 3 years later of pelvic recurrence with involvement of the urinary bladder (obs. DUM).

A careful search of the literature has revealed no published reports of the presence of involved pelvic lymph nodes leading to a diagnosis of carcinoma of the anal canal. Our experience with three such patients, reported on p. 166, is of some interest.

To summarize, late diagnosis is to a certain extent due to the slow development of troublesome symptoms, which delays the patient in seeking medical attention. In addition, some responsibility for delay in performing anorectal digital examination and biopsy can be attributed to the physician who fails to make the correct diagnosis.

One last point that may be mentioned concerns the point of origin of the tumour. The distinction between a squamous cell carcinoma of the anus and an adenocarcinoma of the rectal type is easily made by biopsy in the case of lesions arising from the anorectal junction. But the clinician is able, in most cases, to predict the origin of the lesion. Squamous cell carcinomas tend to infiltrate deeply into underlying structures, and to be annular and so narrow the anal canal, whereas anorectal adenocarcinomas are more ulcerative and exophytic, with raised edges, and do not produce severe narrowing of the anal orifice.

7. Pre-treatment Evaluation

Besides the usual general clinical examination and chest X-ray, the assessment of the spread of a cancer of the anal canal is based on palpation and proctoscopy.

To determine the proximal extent of the lesion, careful digital examination of the anal canal and rectum must be carried out as emphasized previously for rectal cancer, with the patient in the lithotomy position and the knee-chest position. The operator may use the right index finger as well as the left, depending on the site of the lesion.

Combined with anoscopy this examination aims to assess the extent of the tumour around the circumference of the anus, and its upper and lower limits. The length and depth of the lesion and the number of quadrants involved must be recorded. Palpation of the peri-anal area through the intact skin may be helpful, if an indurated edge marking the lateral extent of the tumour is felt.

Digital vagina examination is a great help in defining the upper limit of the growth and the degree of infiltration of the rectovaginal wall. The vaginal mucosa are often stretched by the underlying growth, especially when the tumour is anterior. Invasion of the vaginal mucosa presents as an indurated ulcer situated in the lower half of the vaginal cavity.

If the rectal examination is painful due to narrowing of the anus, ist may be impossible to pass a finger without a general anaesthetic.

A re-examination under general anaesthesia must be carried out in all cases. With relief of pain and relaxation of the sphincter, this is the only way to appreciate the true limits of the tumour, explore the pelvic and perirectal areas, and search for metastatic nodules. As has already been pointed out for cancer of the rectum, metastatic nodes are always indurated; they are situated either in the peri-rectal area (mesenteric lymphatic chain) or on the lateral walls of the pelvis (hypogastric chain), especially in the posterior part of the pelvis. Nodules of venous permeation or in-transit metastasis may be found in the rectovaginal wall as well as in the mesorectum (PAPILLON and BAILLY 1979, PAPILLON et al. 1980).

Metastatic nodules are in most cases situated low down and easily accessible to palpation, as long as it is performed properly. In many cases they appear to be larger than those following rectal cancer, and it is not uncommon to discover two or three metastatic nodes. Needle biopsy of these nodules is often possible by rectal or vaginal approach (Fig. 19).

Thorough inguinal palpation is necessary, especially in the medial part of the groin, as well as the retrocrural area, where external iliac glands may be enlarged. In many cases, the size and the induration of the inguinal nodes give a clear indication of malignancy. However, palpation is not entirely satisfactory in the assessment of inguinal spread, although the superficial inguinal group of lymph nodes is involved first. Lymph nodes enlarged due to inflammation or septic process are usually soft or firm. As has been stressed by GOLIGHER (1975), glands containing malignant deposits are hard. However, doubt may remain about the true nature of the node. In such cases, rather than performing a biopsy and frozen section, the needle biopsy is a very reliable approach to the problem. It is an easy and simple procedure. If carried out with care it gives valid information on the involvement of the inguinal nodes.

At a later stage, there are big, hard, stony masses in the groin, sometimes ulcerated or fixed to underlying structures. The external iliac glands in the retrocrural area may also be enlarged, and palpable above the inguinal ligament.

As far as special investigations are concerned, pedal lymphangiography is helpful in cases with obvious involvement of inguinal nodes in visualizing the external iliac chains and assessing the extent of lymphatic spread beyond the inguinal area. In the case of clinically uninvolved groin, lymphangiography is not necessary, because mesenteric and hypogastric chains are not demonstrated by this method. Liver scan and intravenous pyelography are not part of the usual investigations, but they are necessary in advanced cases. CT scan may be helpful in the detection of pelvic metastatic nodes.

8. Clinical Staging

A common classification of tumours allows comparison of published series and a range of therapeutic procedures. The TNM pretreatment clinical classification (1967) based on clinical, radiological and endoscopic findings, is accepted for most tumours. Applied to carcinomas of the anal canal, the stages are described as follows:

T1 Tumour occupying not more than one-third of the circumference or length of the anal canal, and not infiltrating the external sphincter muscle
T2 Tumour occupying more than one-third of the circumference or length of the anal canal, or infiltrating the external sphincter muscle
T3 Tumour with extension to rectum or skin, but not to other neighbouring structures
T4 Tumour with extension to neighbouring structures

The TNM classification has been criticized on a number of grounds. Firstly, although infiltration of the external sphincter muscle is easily appreciated in an operative specimen, it may be difficult for the clinician to assess. The same case may be classified as T1 by some clinicians, and as T2 by others. Circumferential spread is usually easy to appreciate, while estimation of the length of the tumour is often not accurate enough to be taken as a measure of tumour extension.

Extension to the skin or to the rectum indicates a T3 tumour, but tumours arising from the upper part of the anal canal invade the rectum very soon. In such cases rectal involvement does not mean a bad prognosis. The problem is the same for tumours located below the dentate line. Invasion of the skin of the external margin should not be used as a prognostic factor. Limited tumours, less than 3 cm in diameter, astride the anal canal and involving either the rectum or the skin and classified therefore T3, are cured more easily than T2 tumours involving ¾ of the circumference or infiltrating the sphincter muscle deeply. A last point is that the term neighbouring structures is not precise enough for use in a classification. For these reasons TNM clinical staging has not been adopted by most centres.

Some other classifications have been proposed. In 1970, ROUSSEAU et al. (1973) at the Institut Curie, Paris, suggested that the TNM staging should be modified by introducing the size of the tumour. For example, T3 would be dividet in to:
T3a Tumour less than 4 cm in diameter
T3b Tumour equal to or more than 4 cm in diameter.

At the Centre Léon Bérard a very simple clinical staging based essentially on the size of the tumour has been proposed. This system has been applied to more than 250 cases and has proved effective:

T1　　Tumour not exceeding 2 cm in diamter
T2　　Tumour between 2 cm and 4 cm in diameter
T3　　Tumour larger than 4 cm, mobile, infiltrating neither the vaginal mucosa nor the genito-urinary tract
T4a　Tumour invading the vaginal mucosa
T4b　Tumour with extension to neighbouring structures other than skin, rectum, and vaginal mucosa

From a practical point of view, this classification can be reduced to four groups of cancers involving the anal canal:

T1–T2 Tumours easily controlled
T3　　Tumours which can be controlled possibly with preservation of anal function
T4a　Tumours which can be controlled but with loss of anal function
T4b　Huge and very infiltrating tumours for which curative treatment is unlikely to be possible.

In the majority of published series T1–T2 tumours represent one-third of the lesions, whereas two-thirds of carcinomas of the anal canal are large T3 or T4 tumours at the time of diagnosis.

XI. Treatment

Surgery or radiotherapy may be employed as the first approach to the management of carcinoma of the anal canal. Unfortunately, there has been total disagreement between surgeons and radiotherapists about their respective roles in all but a few institutions. A study of the results of both these methods should allow a comparison of the effectiveness of each technique, and lead to a better understanding of the respective roles of the surgeon and the radiotherapist in the treatment of this type of tumour and the need for a new therapeutic approach.

1. Surgery

a) Local Excision

The simple removal of the growth with a margin of normal tissue, while leaving the rectum and the greater part of the anal canal, has little place in the treatment of carcinoma of the anal canal. There is a discrepancy in the results and the use of this operation, because many reports involve carcinomas of the anal margin and of the anal canal, the delimitations of which are not the same in all institutions.

HOHM and JACKMAN (1964) recommended that all lesions distal to and not involving the dentate line be treated by conservative methods "unless infiltration of the lesion was such that local excision was impossible". They do not specify the degree of infiltration that would preclude it. The survival rate after conservative treatment (18 of 23, 82,6%) supported this view, but it must be emphasized that the majority of the conservatively treated patients also received additive irradiation. They suggest that the increased survival rate of those patients who underwent conservative treatment may have been enhanced by the small size and the low grade of histological malignancy. BEAHRS (1979) reported 31 cases of superficial anal canal cancers treated by local excision, with additive radiation in 15 cases, with a survival rate of 77,7% at 5 years.

HARDCASTLE and BUSSEY (1968) reported eigth cases treated at St. Mark's Hospital between 1928 and 1962 in a series of 127 anal canal cancers, that is 6,2% of cases. Of the eight patients, six survived 5 years; two patients with poorly differentiated tumour developed local recurrence. The author admitted that a local excision seems to be adequate operation only for well-differentiated tumours that are sufficiently small to allow wide removal.

KUEHN et al. (1968) reported a series of 26 cases treated by local excision with 75,2% 5-year survival and two recurrences to the peri-anal region and to the anal canal, which required AP resection.

BEAHRS (1979) published a series of 21 cases with nine (42%) recurrences and a 5-year survival rate of 85%. In the series of STEARNS and QUAN (1970) of 30 cases treated by local excision for lesions of the perineal area or the anal canal, 19 had local recurrences (63%): 11 patients underwent AP or perineal resection; eight had subsequent local excision. Of the 30 patients, 20 (66%) were alive and well at 5 years, but two other patients had late recurrences after 5 years.

PARKS (1981) reported ten patients with squamous lesions of moderate size located in the lower anal canal, treated by local excision and followed up for 3–10 years. There was no recurrence. "As regards to function the only problem has been some difficulty with control of flatus". PARKS mentioned that all these patients were relatively young and he thought that in elderly patients with weak pelvic floor muscles a more severe degree of incontinence might well be encountered. He considered that in such cases radiotherapy and surgery have the same effectiveness.

These figures demonstrate that the selection of the cases suitable for local excision varies from institution to institution. From a review of the literature it can be stated that:

1. All infiltrating tumours are beyond the scope of local excision. Unless an adequate margin can be secured between the growth and the pectinate line, it is unwise to persist with a purely local removal (GOLIGHER 1975). When the size of the tumour would necessitate removal of a large portion of the sphincter muscles which actually renders the patient incontinent, it may be wise to abandon conservative surgical procedure altogether.
2. Some limited pre invasive or slightly invasive carcinomas of the lower part of the anal canal may be treated by local surgery, but postoperative irradiation is advisable in all cases to decrease the incidence of local recurrence, as was suggested by MAC CONNELL (1970) and used by BEAHRS (1979) in 15 of his 36 cases.
3. All cases suitable for local excision are amenable to radiation therapy with a greater chance of local control.
4. There is a possibility of pelvic spread even in early invasive cancer; this is another indication for irradiation either by itself or combined with local excision.
5. It would be erroneous to compare the results of local excision with those of AP resection, because the indications for these operations differ and in many statistics cancers of the lower anal canal and cancers of the anal margin are not distinguished.

b) Major Surgery

Major Surgery is the treatment of choice in the surgical departments of most institutions in western countries. It consists of a radical excision of the rectum and anus, preferably by the AP method. The excision is performed by the same technique as for a cancer of the lower rectum, but with a wide peri-anal and perineal excision to include the levator muscles as well as the contents of the ischiorectal fossae. This wide removal is justified by the presence of cords of neoplastic cells, which may extend for large distances from the anal tumour into the contiguous tissues. In female patients posterior vaginectomy should also be performed if indicated. This leaves an extensive defect, which cannot be closed primarily.

SAWYERS (1972) has described a technique for reconstruction of the vagina after extended AP resection. Gluteal and perineal flaps can be used to replace the resected tissue. These flaps are designed to rebuild the lining of the posterior vagina to the coccyx. This operation removes the whole tumour and the mesenteric lymph nodes, but does not involve the hypogastric nodes. Miles' operation may be extended to include a pelvic lymphadenectomy, as has been described by STEARNS and QUAN (1970).

At the Memorial Sloan Kettering Cancer Center, of the 67 patients who had resections permitting evaluation of the metastasic pelvic iliac lymph nodes, 26 (24%) had metastases to one or more of the nodes. Two patients survived 5 or more years without evidence of recurrence of metastases. Forty-four patients had abdomino-pelvic or extra mesenteric lymphadenectomy in addition to the operation for the primary tumour; 26 were performed at the time of the AP resection and 19 at the time of radical groin dissection: 15 (33%) of these had metastases to the obturator or hypogastric lymph nodes, and five of the 15 (33%) survived 5 or more years. The authors consider that limited dissection of the obturator fossa, and hypogastric area could be done at the time of AP resection without adding to the morbidity, and that some patients with metastases to these nodes can be salvaged. However, this dissection would be technically difficult in markedly obese patients, long narrow male pelves, or where there was excessive pelvic bleeding.

The cure rates for radical excision published in the literature are reported in Table 18. They differ markedly, but the general impression is that the long-term results of surgery for epidermoid carcinoma of the anal canal are usually poorer than those for adenocarcinoma of the rectum. Some authors have suggested preoperative irradiation, either used systematically (NIGRO et al. 1974, QUAN 1978b) or in those patients with suspected invasion of the perineum or perineal soft tissues (CORMAN and HAGGIT 1977) in the belief that such combined procedures result in better chances of cure than radical surgery alone.

Several comments can be made about these results.
1. Major surgery is only applicable to resectable tumours in patients fit for surgery. About 15%–20% of patients with anal canal cancer are not suitable for radical excision and the results of this type of surgery therefore represent the outcome for a selected group of patients.
2. At the Memorial Sloan Kettering Cancer Center, the cure rate has fallen from 57% in 1963 to 33% in 1970, although treatment has been performed by the same surgical team. These results are explained by a larger proportion of advanced cases in the later series (QUAN 1978b), and were the reason for the introduction of a multidisciplinary approach, with a combination of radiotherapy and chemotherapy before surgery, in 1974.
3. The operative mortality rate is higher after surgery for anal cancer than after that for rectal cancer. It may be estimated at between 6% and 8% according to the statistics where operative mortality rate is mentioned (Table 19). In most

Table 18. Results of radical excision (Miles' operation)

Institution or author	No. of cases	5-year survival rate (%)
St. Mark's Hospital, London (HARDCASTLE et al. 1968)	92	48%
Mayo Clinic (BEAHRS 1979, BEAHRS and WILSON 1976)	80	60,7%
Memorial Sloan Kettering Cancer Center, New York (STEARNS and QUAN 1970) 1907–1944	144	41%
1944–1963	109	57%
1963–1970	65	33%
O'BRIEN et al. (1950)	45	31,5%
BOND (1960)	21	43%
DILLARD et al. (1963)	46	58%
KLOTZ et al. (1957)	194	50%
KUEHN et al. (1968)	83	46,8%
SAWYERS (1972)	42	52%
MACCONNELL (1970)	22	42%
BRENNAN and STEWART (1972)	16	37%
LOYGUE et al. (1981)	33	53%
PARADIS et al. (1975)	28	50%
GOLDEN and HORSLEY (1976)	26	54%

Table 19. Mortality rate after Miles' operation for anal cancer

Author	No. of cases	Operation mortality rate
RICHARDS et al. (1962)	61	6,5%
DILLARD et al. (1963)	46	8%
KLOTZ et al. (1967)	19	8,4%
KUEHN et al. (1968)	83	5%
MACCONNELL (1970)	22	8%
PARADIS et al. (1975)	28	4%

series no detail is given about how the survival rate is calculated and whether it is based on operative survivors or on all patients submitted to radical surgery. The figures in Table 19 show that many patients with anal tumour are poor surgical risks.

4. The failures after surgery are usually pelvic or perineal recurrences due to the dissemination of the tumour in the soft tissues or in the lymphatics. Most occur during the first 2 years. They account for 50% of the deaths (SAWYERS 1972). WELCH and MALT (1977) reported 27 recurrences out of 53 patients at a median time for the discovery of 7,5 months after surgery.

5. Although radical excision produces a high cure rate for limited tumours, the chance of survival decreases significantly for patients with large infiltrating tumours and those with involvement of the pelvic nodes. (Table 20). The figures in Table 20 illustrate that lymph node involvement, which is one of the major arguments in favour of radical excision compared with radiation therapy, still has a bad prognostic significance, even after major surgery.

6. Lastly, it must be borne in mind that radical surgery for anal cancer has the same sequelae and complications as for rectal cancer, especially permanent

Table 20. Results of surgery in cases of pelvic nodal involvement

Author	5-year survival rate
Hightower and Tudd (1967)	40%
Beahrs (1979), Beahrs and Wilson (1976)	31,8%
Stearns and Quan (1970)	22%
Corman and Haggitt (1977)	29%
Loygue et al. (1981)	29%

colostomy and genito-urinary troubles, with their psycho-social implications. These complications have been dealt with in Chapter III, which is devoted to rectal cancer.

c) Extended Surgery

Extension to the uterus may require hysterectomy and subtotal vaginectomy, combined with the AP resection. In the male with involvement of the prostate, base of bladder, or seminal vesicles, a pelvic exenteration including cystectomy and construction of an ileobladder might be indicated (Quan 1979).

d) Colostomy

In addition to the colostomy associated with major excisional surgery, colostomies may be needed in several circumstances such as:
1. Severe or complete narrowing of the anal canal with incontinence and obstruction, secondary to large tumours which cannot be resected due to their size or the poor general condition of the patient
2. Failure of radiation therapy in inoperable patients
3. Severe radionecrosis with unbearable pain on defecation.

2. Radiation Therapy

Radiation therapy is the principal method for the conservative treatment of anal canal carcinomas. The aim is to combine control of the disease with preservation of normal anal function without impairment of continence. The tissues of the anal region are known to be very susceptible to high-dose irradiation, with a risk of local necrosis. Many surgeons, especially in the United States, have avoided the use of radiation therapy as the primary treatment of choice for epidermoid carcinoma of the anal canal, because of its failures and its undesirable side-effects, particularly severe radionecrosis (Raven 1941, Gabriel 1941 and Sweet 1947).

Table 21. Statistics from the Institut Curie (COURTIAL and FERNANDEZ COLMEIRO 1960)

Modality of irradiation	No. of cases	5-year survival rate
Radium implant	60	36%
Radium + X-rays (200 kV)	11	9%
X-rays (200 kV)	19	20%
X-rays (500 kV)	83	32,5%
X-rays + radium	10	40%
	183	33,3% (61)

Table 22. Statistics from the Institut Curie (COURTIAL and FERNANDEZ COLMEIRO 1960): 5-year survival rate according to size of tumour

	Tumours < 3 cm	Tumours 3–6 cm	Tumours < 6 cm
5-year survival rate	50%	44%	10%

The first experiences of irradiation of epidermoid cancer of the anal canal date from the 1920s. Since that time, the technique of radiation therapy and our knowledge of the disease have improved in many ways. The purpose of this chapter is to demonstrate that it is now possible to control many large and infiltrating tumours of the anus without a high incidence of complications, provided new protocols of treatment, developed during the last decade, are applied.

a) Historical Backgrounds

A major contribution to the use of irradiation of epidermoid carcinoma of the anal canal was made at the Institut Curie and published in many reports by surgeons and radiotherapists since 1948. After ROUX-BERGER and ENNUYER (1948), COURTIAL and FERNANDEZ COLMEIRO (1960) reported on a series of 183 cases treated between 1921 and 1953. All cases had been followed up for over 5 years. According to the period of time and to the extent of the tumour, several procedures have been applied. The results are presented in Table 21.

Of the 61 patients who survived 5 years, 50 (27%) were treated by irradiation alone, 11 had subsequent surgery for failure or necrosis. All deaths were included, whatever their cause. Most patients had large tumours; 36% had tumours bigger than 6 cm and were given palliative irradiation. Only 20% had tumours which did not exceed 3 cm. The chance of cure is correlated with the size of the lesion (Table 22).

In the interpretation of these results, it must be emphasized that this series represents the most extensive experience of irradiation of carcinoma of the anal canal before the era of supervoltage radiation therapy, and that these statistics span a long period of time, starting in 1921 at the dawn of the use of radium needles and dosimetry. This explains why among the 61 cured patients, 15 had major complications, severe radionecrosis or fibrous stenosis necessitating an iliac colostomy, so that the functional results fell short of expectation. This complication was almost exclusively one of interstitial radium, and the authors abandoned radium in favor of high-voltage roentgen rays (500 kV) for extensive growths. However, it may be pointed out that in the group of patients with limited or moderately advanced tumour, the cure rate was 36,3%.

In the 1960s the first publications concerning the use of cobalt therapy stressed the decrease in the incidence of radionecrotic complications. However, most surgeons remained convinced that radiotherapy should only be employed for patients with locally inoperable growths or whose general conditions would make major surgery particularly hazardous. There were several reasons for the reluctance of surgeons to refer their patients for irradiation at this time:
1. Radiation therapy was reserved for patients with advanced tumour which could not be cured by other means.
2. Many radiotherapists treated squamous cell carcinomas of the anal canal in the same way as squamous cell carcinomas of other locations in spite of the great differences in the radiation response of the tumour and the soft tissues of the perineum.
3. The modalities of irradiation available in the 1950s were radium implant and orthovoltage X-ray therapy. Neither of these methods adapted well to the management of large anal cancers.

An example of this situation is given by WILLIAMS (1962), who reported on a series of 35 patients treated at St. Bartholomew's Hospital, London, 32 by high-voltage X-ray beam (1 MeV) and three by radium implant. All these patients were considered inoperable. There were twelve 5-year survivors free of disease but in seven cases colostomies were necessary for anal stricture, rectovaginal fistula, or radionecrosis. In another review of 77 cases collected from the literature by GOLDEN and HORSLEY (1976) the 5-year survival rate after radiotherapy was 26%.

From 1955 up to the last decade, two principal methods of irradiation have been applied to epidermoid carcinoma of the anal canal: interstitial curietherapy and external beam irradiation with cobalt-60.

b) Interstitial Curietherapy

Interstitial curietherapy, whatever the radioactive element used, is a technique applicable only to limited and well-defined target volumes. It gives high-dose irradiation over a short period of time with satisfactory protection of the surrounding structures. If the method is applied to large tumours, it produces a high incidence of radionecrotic complications.

During the past 30 years many authors have reported small groups of patients treated by radium implant, but there are very few series with numbers large enough to enable judgement of the effectiveness of the method. For instance in 1960 DEVOIS and DECKER from Paris reported on a series of 21 patients treated by radium in volume implant, with primary control of 14. Of 13 patients followed up for 4–7 years, nine were cured (Table 23). The failures were related to the upward spread of the tumour and to lymphatic spread. Radionecrosis was observed in five patients, and required a definitive colostomy in three and a temporary colostomy in two. The most useful information can derived from the series of the Christie Hospital, Manchester, and the Centre Léon Bérard, Lyon.

Statistics from the Christie Hospital. In 1961, DALBY and POINTON published a series of 171 cases of anal carcinoma treated from 1932 to 1955. Thirty-four cases (20%) were considered to be so advanced that no useful treatment was possible; 31 cases (18%) were referred for surgery, and 106 cases (62%) were treated by interstitial irradiation with radium needles. One hundred and thirty tumours were located in the anal canal and 41 at the anal margin. For small lesions limited to one side of the anal canal, a single-plane implant was employed, aiming at a dose of 6000 rad over 7 days. For thicker lesions, a two-plane implant was necessary. The dose did not exceed 5 500 rad in 7 days.

Of the 59 patients with anal canal carcinoma followed up over 5 years, 23 were alive and well. The 5-year survival rate was 39%. According to the size of the lesion, the 5-year survival rate was 59% for early or moderately advanced tumours, and 20% for late lesions. Ten patients developed a necrosis of a serious nature, six requiring colostomy and four radical excision. Thirteen other patients developed less severe necrosis. The authors concluded that for early and moderately advanced lesions, radium implantation provides a satisfactory method of treatment, whereas more advanced lesions gave very poor results after irradiation and were referred for surgery or were considered as unsuitable for any form of treatment.

Statistics from the Centre Léon Bérard (PAPILLON (1974) PAPILLON et al. (1979, 1980). Between 1949 and 1970, the usual method of irradiation was interstitial radium therapy. Eighty-eight patients were treated: 58 had limited tumours smaller than 4 cm, 30 had tumours equal to or larger than 4 cm in diameter. Selection of the cases suitable for radium implant was performed and the most infiltrating tumours were referred for surgery in the same way as the Christie Hospital series. During the first period between 1949 and 1962, radium implant was performed in one stage. Since 1963, fractionation was often used in order to increase the chance of control in cases of rather large tumours without increasing the incidence of severe radionecrosis. Radium needles 4 cm long containing 4 mg radium were used. The majority of interstitial treatment consisted of volume implants, although one-plane implants for small lesions were sometimes performed. When curietherapy was carried out in one stage, the dose delivered to the target volume was moderate – about 4000 to 5000 rad over 3–4 days.

In the case of fractionated curietherapy, the first implant was directed to the periphery of the tumour at the junction between neoplastic tissue and normal tissue. The dose delivered was 4000 rad at the margin of the lesion, and only 1 500 or 2 000 rad at the centre of the tumour. This very inhomogeneous dose proved to be very efficient, and the shrinkage of many tumours was striking some weeks later. The second stage of radium implant took place 8 weeks after the first and was directed to the residual lesion at the centre of the initial tumour volume. A dose of 2 500–3 000 rad was delivered over 2–3 days. The fractionation technique proved to be very informative in showing the slow regression of the anal tumours and the possibility of taking advantage of this feature to give a higher chance of cure in patients with large tumours. In this situation, radium needles can never be implanted in an ideal spatial arrangement with satisfactory parallelism. The usual arrangement produces hot spots of high-dose radiation, whereas other parts receive much lower doses.

Of the 88 patients treated and followed up over 5 years, 60 patients were alive and disease-free at 5 years (68%). Severe radionecrosis was observed in 5% of cases. Benign ulcerative reaction resolving spontaneously in less than 3 months, without sequelae, was observed in a high percentage (45%) of cases. Of these 60 patients who had survived at 5 years, 53 had been treated exclusively by radium needling, seven after subsequent surgery for failures (four cases) or necrosis (three cases). Twenty-eight patients died before 5 years: 15 (17%) from cancer; 12 from intercurrent disease, the anal cancer being locally controlled; one post-operatively after failure. Of 15 patients who died of cancer, two died of distant metastasis. It must be added that among the 60 5-year survivors, three died of cancer after 9, 12, and 13 years respectively, two of regional failures and one of metastases. Twelve local failures (14%) were observed: only two were controlled after surgery. Ten patients died.

The incidence of local failures varies according to the type of curietherapy. After one stage of curietherapy in 33 patients, eight failures were observed (25%), whereas in 55 patients treated with fractionated curietherapy in two stages separated by 2 months, the rate of local failure dropped to 8%, although the number of large tumours was higher in this group. Fourteen patients developed pelvic lymph node recurrences, e.i. metastases in the pararectal lymphnodes or in the iliac or sacral nodes. Eight patients died from cancer before 5 years. Six patients have had their disease controlled for more than 5 years. two after AP resection, four after interstitial curietherapy of the pararectal node. One of the two patients clinically controlled after radical surgery developed an inguinal metastasis in the 6th year and died from cancer. All the other patients are still alive or died from intercurrent disease, locally controlled.

Curietherapy was abandoned in 1970 in favour of an association of external irradiation and interstitial curietherapy in a split course. In conclusion, interstitial curietherapy can control quite a high percentage of limited anal canal tumours, but the principal criticisms which can be made of this method are:
1. The high incidence of painful reactions and necrosis
2. The rate of local and, above all, nodal failures related to the treatment of limited target volume, which does not include the pelvic drainage areas.

Table 23. Anal canal carcinoma: Statistical data for interstitial curietherapy with radium

Author	No. of cases	5-year survival rate	Rate of severe necrosis
Devois and Decker (1960), Paris	13	69%	23%
Dalby and Pointon (1961), Manchester	59	39%	10%
Papillon (1974) and Papillon et al. (1973, 1979), Lyon	88	68%	5%

Of the 60 survivors, three died of cancer in the 9th, 12th and 13th years.

c) External Beam Irradiation with Cobalt-60

Two detailed accounts of the use of external beam irradiation have been published, by the Institut Curie. Paris, and by the Institut Gustave Roussy, Villejuif (France). The techniques used were different, but all patients were treated with gamma rays of cobalt-60, and never with high-energy electrons. It has been stated that severe skin reactions and high rates of complications occur in patients treated by electrons, and this type of irradiation beam is not indicated as a definitive treatment in cases of carcinoma of the anal canal.

Statistics from the Institut Curie. PILLERON (1973) ROUSSEAU et al. (1979) published the long-term results of a series of 128 squamous cell carcinomas of the anal canal treated by radical teletherapy with cobalt. Two protocols of irradiation were used:

Protocol 1. A dose of 6000–7000 rad was delivered to the anal area over 8–9 weeks by a perineal field 8×8 cm or 10×10 cm. The size of the fields was reduced to 6×6 cm after a dose of 6000 rad had been distributed. Irradiation of the inguinal areas was performed to a given dose of 6000 rad. This protocol was applied to limited tumours located below the dentate line. Of 51 patients with lesions smaller than 4 cm in diameter, 39 (68%) were alive and disease-free at 5 years.

Protocol 2. The target volume encompassed the whole pelvis, the anal area, and the groins. Five fields were used:
one anterior pelvic field, including the inguinal areas
one posterior pelvic field, including the anus. A dose of 4500–5000 rad mid-line of the pelvis was delivered by these portals. A booster dose of up to 6000 rad was given using:
two inguinal fields
one direct perineal field

This protocol was applied to lesions larger than 4 cm or located above the dentate line. Of 71 patients treated in such a way, 22 (32%) were alive and well at 5 years.

Statistics from the Institut Gustave Roussy. ESCHWEGE et al. (1979) reported a series of 138 patients treated exclusively with external irradiation. Thirty-two patients did not receive complete irradiation and were therefore excluded from the analysis. Cobalt-60 was applied through arc-therapy of 240° focused on the ano-rectal area, the patient being in the prone position. The target volume encompassed the anal canal and the lymphatic drainage areas of the posterior part of the pelvis. It had the shape of a cylinder 10–15 cm long and 6–9 cm in diameter. A tumour dose of 6500 rad was given over 6 weeks. The 5-year survival rates were 62% for limited tumours and 26% for large tumours, with a high incidence of major complications (Table 24).

Comments. These reports show that external irradiation with cobalt-60 can control a large number of limited cancers of the anal canal, but does not give satisfac-

Table 24. Results of external beam irradiation with cobalt-60

	No. of cases	5-year survival rate (disease-free)
Institut Curie (ROUSSEAU et al. 1979)	128	48%
T ≤ 4 cm	57	68%
T > 4 cm	71	32%
Institut Gustave Roussy (ESCHWEGE et al. 1979)	106	42%
T ≤ 4 cm		62%
T > 4 cm		26%

tory results for infiltrating tumours larger than 4 cm. In addition, the danger of severe necrosis is so great that this method cannot be considered the optimal procedure for such lesions, which represent a substantial proportion of anal canal cancers. For instance, in the series reported by ROUSSEAU et al. (1979) and by ESCHWEGE et al. (1979) the rates of severe radionecrosis were 20% and 34% respectively. In the latter series only 25 of 106 patients were cured without impairment of anal function.

To summarize, it may be concluded that the usual modalities of radiation therapy are not well adapted to the conservative treatment of large tumours of the anal canal, which represent the majority of cases of anal canal cancer at the time of diagnosis, and that it is necessary to define new protocols of irradiation.

d) Complications of Irradiation

The main objection to irradiation of carcinoma of the anal canal is the risk of severe complications occuring after application of high-dose radiation to the anal region. The tissues irradiated are highly prone to necrosis, but the frequency of complications and the degree and extent of damage to perineal structures depend on three basic factors:
1. The extent of the disease and of the infiltrated area are significant. Radionecrosis is less common in limited cancers than in advanced, ulcerative, and infiltrating tumours, which have involved large areas of sphincter muscle and peri-anal soft tissues such as the rectovaginal wall.
2. The risk is greater in the elderly and in patients with loss of weight, arteriosclerosis, and poor circulation than in robust, middle-aged patients.
3. The danger of radionecrotic complications is closely related to the modalities of irradiation. Dose, volume, and time are the key factors in the pathogenesis of necrosis. The technique and the schedule of radiation play a large part in the successful conservation of anal function. This problem is the responsibility of the radiotherapist, who must take great care in the selection of the most appropriate procedure and in planning treatment of each individual patient.

There are two types of complication:
- benign reactions or sequelae, which are easily tolerated
- severe radionecrosis, which alters the quality of life and represents a major complication.

Benign Complications. Superficial mucosal ulceration of the anal canal may be responsible for local pain and discomfort some weeks following irradiation. A temporary colostomy is never required, as skin and mucosal reactions are transient and usually settle spontaneously or with simple measures such as ointment and analgesics, and the patient recovers an entirely normal anal function without untoward effects.

Telangiectasia of the peri-anal skin and/or a slight fibrosis of the anal canal cannot be regarded as severe complications as long as they do not result in discomfort, but they may be prevented by using appropriate treatment schedules. Telangiectasia of the rectal mucosa may give rise to occasional bleeding and even to anaemia. They are easily controlled by local applications of chromic acid (one-third strength), or steroid enemas. All these complications are compatible with a normal life.

Major Complications. Major Complications depend on the method of irradiation, and consist either of severe radionecrosis or significant fibrosis. Severe radionecrosis presents as a sloughing ulceration excavating the anal area, at times associated with rectovaginal fistula. The pain is constant and unbearable, and exacerbated by defecation. It gives rise to an extreme discomfort with a serious influence on the psychological and physical balance of the patient. This complication starts a few months after irradiation, never after the 1 year, and may be observed after interstitial curietherapy as well as after cobalt therapy. It lasts a very long time, with no tendency to spontaneous healing, and medical treatment fails to improve the condition of the patient, so that most patients require a colostomy and, in some cases, a perineal resection. Severe radionecrosis may be associated with treatment failure, and the biopsy which alone could assess the presence of neoplastic tissue in the vicinity of the ulceration may be delayed by the fear of worsening the radionecrosis. Cytology may be helpful in such cases.

Significant fibrotic dystrophy of the peri-anal area is only observed after high doses of external irradiation. Electron beams have been proscribed in the treatment of anal canal tumours because of the unacceptably high risk of radiodystrophy. This complication consists of fibrous stenosis of the anal canal, with incontinence, narrowing of the urethra in males, oedema of the vulva or of the penis and fibrosis of the perineal soft tissues, giving rise to discomfort in the sitting position. This type of complication, related to the large target volume irradiated, may occur rather late – up to the 3rd year. ROUSSEAU et al. 1973 reported that severe fibrosis may develop between 3 months and 3 years after completion of external irradiation with cobalt-60: 60% in the 1st year, 20% in the 2nd, and 20% in the 3rd year. In the series from the Institut Curie, ROUSSEAU et al. (1973) mentioned that only 35% of the cured patients were free of major complications, and that of the 15 cases of severe radionecrosis, 13 were observed in patients who had received a dose of cobalt-60 higher than 7000 rad.

XII. New Therapeutic Approaches

1. Background

In many institutions, radiation therapy has been reserved for patients with lesions considered to be incurable or beyond resection by radical surgery. This approach is not a valid test of the effectiveness of irradiation in the management of more favourable lesions.

It is time to draw attention to the progress that has been made in irradiation of anal canal cancer, and to reconsider the response of this tumour to irradiation.

Squamous cell carcinoma of the anal canal has its own individual character, and should not be irradiated as squamous carcinomas of other locations, such as carcinomas of the tongue, pharynx, or uterine cervix.

There are several reasons why anal canal carcinoma requires specific techniques of irradiation.

a) Accessibility

The upper and lower limits of the tumour are easy to assess. Most sites of lymphatic involvement can be reached by the examining finger if clinical examination is done with care. The opportunity to palpate the whole tumour and the early sites of lymphatic involvement must be stressed, because this procedure permits assessment of the tumour volume at any time, before, during, and after irradiation. Shrinkage of the tumour and of the nodes may be appreciated, as well as the quality of the scar. Cytology may also be of some help, either by study of scrape smears from the site of the tumour, or by aspiration biopsy of the inguinal and pelvic nodes. Moreover, endocurietherapy is possible because these tumours are easy to reach. The role of curietherapy is well known, and accepted as a definitive procedure for local control of many squamous cancers, including the tongue and the uterine cervix, and therefore may be useful for anal canal tumours. It would be unreasonable not to take advantage of the possibility of using it in the treatment of tumours of the anal canal.

b) Radiosensitivity

Epidermoid carcinoma of the anal canal is highly radiosensitive. It is more radiosensitive than it is usually thought to be, and more so than most squamous cancers arising from other mucosa. This property can be appreciated by the study of the shrinkage of the lesion and its disappearance at clinical examination, as well as by the control of the disease as judged from examination of the operative specimen, and from cured patients who have been treated by irradiation alone.

The response to radiotherapy is not limited to the primary tumour, and is seen in inguinal and pelvic metastatic nodes. It is probably related to the poor histological differentiation of most tumours, including basaloid or cloacogenic carcinomas, as well as squamous tumours. This conclusion is drawn from a series of 246 cases treated by irradiation at the Centre Léon Bérard. In this series there were no muco-epidermoid carcinomas, which are less radiosensitive.

There is, however, a small percentage of tumours of no specific histological type which will not be controlled by irradiation. These lesions are apparently identical to those that do respond, from both the gross and microscopic points of view.

To summarize, the susceptibility of most epidermoid carcinomas of the anal canal to irradiation is not well recognized in many institutions, which consider radiation therapy as a palliative procedure applicable only to advanced and inoperable tumours. The response justifies a more privileged place for radiation therapy in the management of this type of tumour.

c) Radionecrosis

Severe radionecroses are generally due to overdosage, to faulty technique, or to wrongly adapted protocol of irradiation applied to large infiltrating tumours. They are the responsibility of the radiotherapist, who must bear in mind that there is a narrow margin between local failure due to underdosage and severe radionecroses due to overdosage. The choice of an optimal protocol of irradiation is decisive in all cases submitted to exclusive irradiation for cure. Whatever the purpose (radical or pre-operative irradiation), the tolerance of perineal structures should always be taken into consideration.

d) Time Factor

The most peculiar problem of squamous anal canal carcinoma is its slow "evolutive tempo". It is well known that this type of tumour grows slowly and that it takes many months to reach appreciable volume, but one of the most surprising and overlooked characteristics is its slow rate of regression after irradiation. Usually there is an obvious reduction in the tumour volume after irradiation of squamous cancer at a dose of 4000 rad over 4 weeks, which allows endocurietherapy to be performed in the first few days after completion of the irradiation for patients with cervical cancer or oropharyngeal cancer.

With anal canal carcinoma, the pace of shrinkage differs markedly from that with cervical and oropharyngeal tumours. After irradiation of a large tumour at a dose of 3000 rad or 4000 rad over 3 weeks, there is almost no immediate shrinkage, and the tumour volume at the completion of treatment is almost the same as it was at the beginning. Size, consistency, and degree of infiltration of the tumour into the surrounding tissues will not have changed substantially. This delayed response can be misinterpreted as a sign of radioresistance, and may lead to endocurietherapy to the entire tumour volume, with disastrous results.

In fact, the size of the tumour is not reduced by more than half at 1 month after completion of the irradiation. The shrinkage will continue during the 2th month, at the end of which it appears most marked. Even when the lesion was very large, it will often have been reduced to a small residual tumour by this time and clinical examination may indicate that it has disappeared entirely. In the experience at the Centre Léon Bérard, no tumour extension has been observed during this period. The end of the 2th month is the best time to perform the endocurietherapy, which is applied as a booster dose to a reduced tumour volume.

This split-course treatment with a long interval aims to allow the normal tissues time to recover, and to reduce the danger of radionecrosis with a greater chance of local control. This important time factor used in the irradiation of squamous cell carcinoma of the anal canal differs from the protocol used for other squamous tumours and is vital for proper treatment of this type of tumour.

e) Multimodality Treatment

Many trials have been conducted in the United States and in Europe to try to enhance the effectiveness of radiotherapy by using radiosensitizers or chemical drugs such as bleomycin, methotrexate, or fluorouracil. The purpose of such combined methods is to obtain the same biological effect with a lower dose of radiation, and so with a lower risk of complications. In the particular case of carcinoma of the anal canal, the danger of major necrosis after high-dose radiation encourages the radiotherapist to use several modes of treatment to increase the chance of control of the disease without inducing a high rate of severe radionecrosis.

2. Recent Developments

During the past 10 years, substantial changes have occurred in the approach to the management of epidermoid carcinoma of the anal canal. All publications emphasize the need for irradiation to play a major role, and the trend is to abandon surgery as the only treatment for all cases. There are two new approaches:
1. Pre-operative irradiation with or without chemotherapy, which has been initiated in the United States and in France
2. Split-course irradiation taking advantage of the slow pace of the shrinkage of anal canal tumours after irradiation. This modality has been developed in Moscow and especially in Lyon.

a) Pre-operative Irradiation With or Without Chemotherapy

Failures of radical surgery for large tumours have already been emphasized, and more and more attention is being paid to the usefulness of a pre-surgical approach.

Preoperative Radiochemotherapy. The most significant work has been conducted in Detroit and in New York City. In 1973 NIGRO et al. (1974, 1981) at a meeting of the American Proctologic Society, gave a preliminary report, "Combined Therapy for Cancer of the Anal Canal". Disappointed by the results of major surgery, the authors published the cases of three patients with biopsy-proven, primary operable epidermoid carcinoma of the anal canal, treated by a combined pre-surgical approach consisting of:
1. External irradiation: 3000 rad mid-line to the pelvis and anus over a 3-week period by two opposed fields.
2. Chemotherapy: 5-fluorouracil (5-FU) 25 mg/kg body wt daily in 5% glucose in the form of a continous 24-hour infusion for 5 days, starting on day 1 of the radiation therapy, and also mitomycin C (MTC) 0,5 mg/kg body wt as a single bolus injection on the 1st day.

Abdominoperineal resection of the rectum was performed 6 weeks later in two of the three patients. No tumour was found in the operative specimens, and the patients were well 14 and 6 months later. The third patient refused operation and was well 4 months later.

Stimulated by these preliminary results, NIGRO et al. (1981) updated this series, and reported the cases of 19 patients treated in the same manner. Following radiation and chemotherapy, there was no evidence of gross tumour in 15 patients. In the other four patients, the tumour decreased at least 50% in size. Twelve of the 19 patients had AP resections. The specimens were clear of tumour cells in seven and contained only microscopic tumour in one, and in four tumour was gross and microscopic. Seven of the 19 patients treated more recently, whose lesions disappeared macroscopically, had wide excision of the scar. There was no microscopic tumour in any of these specimens; radical surgery was not performed. Eleven patients were alive and well, disease-free, for 3–7 years; five died from cancer. NIGRO et al. (1981) concluded that some patients may be spared AP resection when treated in the manner described.

At the Memorial Sloan Kettering Cancer Centre the same policy has been applied to 26 patients with anal canal squamous-cell carcinoma since 1974. This is the most important series published in the United States. The results were reported in publications by NEWMAN and QUAN (1976), by QUAN (1979) and QUAN et al. (1978). QUAN (1979) using the same protocol, emphasized the rapid and impressive shrinkage of the tumour in most cases (25 of 26), the high rate of tumour-free operative specimens (14 of 26), and the possibility of local surgical procedures instead of the AP resection necessary if these patients had been treated by exclusive surgery. The more conservative approach, i.e. the excisional biopsy of the bed of the lesion in a full-thickness fashion, was "considered feasible, because of the dramatic gross disappearance of the tumour following chemotherapy and radiotherapy".

WANEBO et al. (1980, 1981) published a contribution to the multimodality approach to the surgical management of locally advanced epidermoid carcinoma of the anorectum. They reported a series of seven patients, which can be divided into two groups. Three patients with recurrent or persistent disease previously treated either by radium implant (two) or by AP resection (one) received chemotherapy (5-FU, MTC) 3–8 weeks before surgery. Tumour regression due to chemotherapy was greater than 50% in one patient and between 25% and 50% in another, and no regression was observed in the third. Four patients previously untreated had a pre-surgical approach based on irradiation (3 000 rad in 3 weeks) and chemotherapy (5-FU, MTC). Tumour regression was greater than 50% in all cases and complete in one case (no tumour found in the operative specimen). Two of these patients, in spite of the very advanced lesion, were alive and well, disease-free, more than 2 years after treatment. It was concluded that combined pre-operative radiochemotherapy gives patients with locally advanced carcinoma of the anal canal a better chance of cure than surgery alone.

CUMMINGS et al. (1980) reported on preliminary results obtained in six patients with carcinoma of the anal canal, treated by irradiation combined with chemotherapy (5-FU, MTC) at the Princess Margaret Hospital, Toronto, between May 1978 and August 1979. Radical radiotherapy was applied to the primary tumour (5 000 rad over 4 weeks), and to the inguinal and pelvic lymph nodes (3 000 rad in 2½ weeks). In all six patients local tumour control was achieved and anal continence retained.

In 1979, BRUCKNER et al. at the Mount Sinai-Hospital, New York, reported three cases of recurrent squamous cell carcinoma of the anus following failure of attempted curative resections (two AP resections, one local excision), which were treated by chemotherapy and radiotherapy, and in which the tumours were controlled locally by this combined approach. BRUCKNER et al. (1979) mentioned that "in the dosages used (3 000 rads in 3 weeks) radiotherapy alone was very unlikely to have produced the results observed in his patients and that similarly, 5-FU infusion, with complete remissions". It seems that the favourable results obtained by the association of radiotherapy and chemotherapy are due to an additive or more likely to a synergetic effect, although it will be demonstrated in the next chapter that such results may be obtained by irradiation alone, as long as sophisticated methods of irradiation are applied.

Pre-operative Irradiation Without Chemotherapy. LOYGUE et al. (1981) reported on a series of 132 patients treated either by surgery, by combined radiotherapy and surgery, or by definitive irradiation. The overall 3-year survival rate was 67%. They pointed out that of patients with large infiltrating tumours, the 3-year survival rate after pre-operative irradiation and subsequent AP resection was 50%. They emphasized the advantage of postponing surgery for 1–3 months after completion of the irradiation, and suggested that radical surgery alone be abandoned in favour of irradiation at a dose of 4 000 rad over 4 weeks. After a while the decision was taken either to carry on irradiation up to 6 500 rad in cases of substantial shrinkage of the lesion, or to perform radical resection in cases of significant residual tumour.

SVENSON and MONTAGUE (1980) reported 24 cases of transitional cloacogenic carcinoma of the anus treated with curative intent by AP resection alone (15 patients), combination AP resection and irradiation (six patients), and irradiation alone (three patients). Surgery alone failed to control disease in seven of 15 patients. No local and pelvic failures occurred in patients treated with irradiation alone or pre-operative or post-operative irradiation. They emphasized the need for radiotherapy to play a major role in the treatment of the tumour. In a recent paper PARKS (1981) shared the same opinion. He thought that for tumours of the upper anal canal "it would seem reasonable that, one should firstly treat with radiotherapy and assess the effectiveness of it. Manifestly if the tumor does not disappear completely, then surgery is essential. If healing is complete however, then careful follow-up will be necessary, particularly in the two years after treatment". He added that among surgeons "there is a considerable resistance to radiotherapy in this area and one has to ask why this should be".

These series deserve a special attention when one takes into consideration that:

1. This change in the policy in the management of epidermoid carcinoma has been worked out by surgical teams who had had long experience in the major surgery applied to this tumour and who were disappointed by the poor long-term results after radical excision in cases of advanced but operable tumour (5-year survival rate: 33% at the Memorial Hospital).
2. Many patients given combined treatment for local control had large, very infiltrating tumours of the anal canal with or without inguinal involvement. The presence of metastatic nodes in the groin was compatible with control of the disease, whereas this sign is usually thought to have a very poor prognostic significance.
3. Considering these data, the authors are encouraged to do more local excision for cure whenever feasible, rather than doing AP resection for this disease. They are even wondering if some patients could be spared surgery completely.

In spite of the rather short follow-up time for most cases and the necessity of a continued experience to determine the efficacy of this new approach, it must be borne in mind that in cases of epidermoid carcinoma of the anal canal treated by surgery or radiotherapy, most failures occur during the first 2 years following treatment, and that the recent reports deserve particular attention.

To summarize, it is admitted that a first approach by radiotherapy, possibly combined with chemotherapy, and followed or not according to the situation by surgery, gives patients a better chance of cure than radical surgery alone.

b) Split-course Irradiation

Split-course irradiation aims to take advantage of the particularly slow shrinkage of anal tumours after irradiation to prevent damage to normal structures, and to adapt the dose required to eradicate the tumours to its own radiosensitivity (Fig. 20). Most of this work has been conducted in two centres: Hospital 57, Moscow; and the Centre Léon Bérard, Lyon.

Experience at Hospital 57. MOSCOW CHRUSCOV et al. (1978) have applied a split-course irradiation to 66 patients with epidermoid carcinoma located in 47 cases in the anal canal and in 19 cases at the anal margin. The tumours were inoperable either because of tumour spread (50), or because of refusal of radical therapy (16). Split-course irradiation was used in order to test the radiosensitivity of each tumour. The first stage consisted of a gamma-ray therapy which gave a focal dose of 4000–4500 rad over 3 weeks, through fixed fields and/or through rotational therapy. A 3-week rest period followed. The procedure of irradiation used in the second stage depended on the degree of shrinkage of the tumour. When the tumour had clinically disappeared, a second course of gamma-ray therapy was given to deliver a booster dose of 2000–2500 rad. When there was a small and flat residual lesion, intracavitary radiation therapy with axial radioactive applicator was used (35 cases). When the residual tumour was large, radical surgery (nine cases) or palliative irradiation was carried out. The 3-year survival rate was 56,3% and the 5-year survival rate 44%. Only one patient required a colostomy for radionecrosis. A minor late complication consisted of skin atrophy, with telangiectasia, dryness, and tenderness of the rectal mucosa, but anal function could be maintained by careful regulation of defecation. Two patients had late-onset haemorrhagic rectitis, which was controlled by conservative means.

XIII. Experience at the Centre Léon Bérard

(PAPILLON 1976, PAPILLON and GERARD 1975, PAPILLON et al. 1980)

Several reports have shown that when surgery is the only means of treatment applied to resectable tumours, the cure rate is high for limited tumours. However, this figure does not exceed 40% when the tumours are large and there is lymphatic spread.

Experience with external irradiation at the Institut Curie and Institut Gustave Roussy has shown that this method will control a small number of large T_3 infiltrating tumours, which, as a group, represent 60% of anal canal cancers.

The use of interstitial curietherapy (PAPILLON 1974) at the Centre Léon Bérard has demonstrated that:
1. High-dose irradiation is not always necessary, and in most cases moderate dosage results in control of limited tumours with a low rate of severe complications.
2. Fractionation increases the effectiveness of irradiation for large, infiltrating tumours and improves the tolerance of perineal structures.
3. Nodal pelvic failures after purely local treatment are so common that this problem must be taken into consideration in all cases, even in early cancer, so that purely local therapy for anal canal cancer, by curietherapy or by cobalt-60, should be proscribed in favour of a systematic treatment of the main lymphatic drainage areas in the pelvis.

Cases of squamous cell carcinoma of the anal canal differ markedly according to the condition of the patient, the stage of the disease, and the presence or absence of regional spread. There is no one single policy adapted to these various problems. It is illogical to deal with so many presentations by single approach, whether surgical or radiotherapeutic. It is therefore necessary to design several protocols of treatment, taking into consideration the substantial progress which has been made in the irradiation of this tumour.

Patients with carcinoma of the anal canal can be divided into two groups: those with resectable tumours, who could be theoretically, treated by surgery with a curative purpose; and those with unresectable tumours, who are not suitable for radical surgery. The first group must be divided into two subgroups: (a) patients considered suitable for curative treatment with preservation of anal sphincter; and (b) patients suitable for curative treatment but without preservation of anal sphincter. In accordance with these data three protocols have been used at the Centre Léon Bérard since 1971:

First protocol: Combination of external irradiation and interstitial curietherapy in a split course
Second protocol: Pre-operative irradiation followed by radical surgery
Third protocol: Whole-pelvic and perineal irradiation.

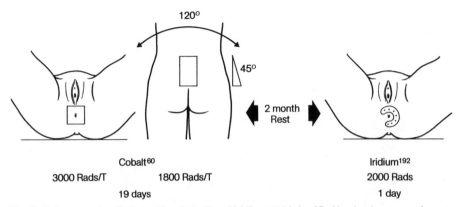

Fig. 20. Split-course irradiation with cobalt-60 and iridium-192 is justified by the slow regression rate of anal canal epidermoid carcinoma. The moderate dosage of irradiation used aims to reduce the incidence of radionecrosis

1. First Protocol – Association of Cobalt-60 and Iridium-192 Implant in a Split Course

The first protocol consists of two stages separated by a free interval of 2 months. Since 1971 it has been applied to 151 patients with tumours that seemed to be suitable for a curative and conservative treatment.

First Stage: External Beam Irradiation by Cobalt-60. Two fields are used. Through a direct perineal field 8 × 8 cm a tumour dose of 3000 rad calculated at 5 cm is delivered in ten fractions within 16 days (Fig. 20). The beam is angled 10° downwards. The given dose at the surface is 4200 rad. Irradiation of the perineal field is made with the patient in the lithotomy position with buttocks taped apart.

Since 1974, irradiation of the presacral area has been added, so that the main lymphatic drainage areas are encompassed in the target volume. Presacral irradiation is applied using arc therapy (120° with a 45° wedge filter through a field 7 × 12 cm, the lower limit of which is situated 7 cm above the anal verge). This irradiation gives a depth dose of 1800 rad at 8 cm in six fractions. Thanks to the combined action of perineal and sacral fields, the minimum tumour dose in the anal and presacral area is 3000 rad. The overall treatment time is 19 days (Fig. 21).

After this first sequence of treatment, there is an interval of 2 months before application of the iridium implant. This long free interval is well adapted to the

Fig. 21. First stage of split-course regimen: Isodose distribution of irradiation with cobalt-60 through two fields. Through a perineal field *(1)* 8 × 8 cm, a dose of 3000 rad calculated at 5 cm depth is delivered in ten fractions over 16 days. The beam is angled 10° downwards on the horizontal line. Through a sacral field *(2)* 7 × 12 cm irradiation, using arc therapy 120° with a 45° wedge filter, a dose of 1800 rad at 8 cm is given in six fractions. The lower limit of the sacral field is 7 cm above the anal verge. Overall treatment time is 19 days. A minimum dose of 3000 rad is given to a target volume encompassing the anal canal, the lower rectum, and most of the pelvic lymphatic drainage areas up to S_1

First Protocol

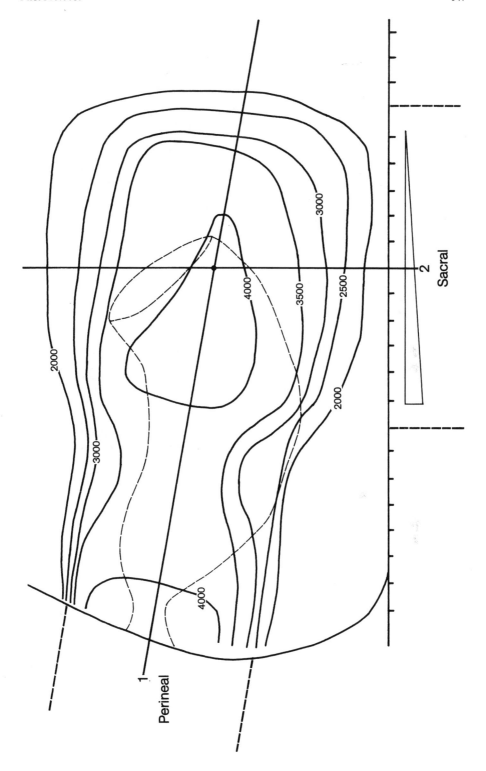

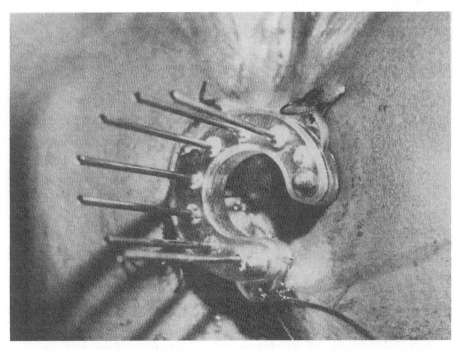

Fig. 22. One-plane iridium-192 implant is carried out 2 months after completion of cobalt therapy. A plastic template with a series of holes 0.9 cm apart is sutured to the peri-anal skin. Seven steel needles are inserted. They will receive the 5-cm-long iridium wires. The dose delivered is 2000 rad

slow regression of squamous cell carcinoma of the anal canal. One must emphasize that at the end of cobalt therapy there is almost no shrinkage of the tumour. One month later the reduction in size is substantial, but there is further regression during the next 4 weeks. In many cases, even in cases of large tumours exceeding 4 cm, there is no clinical evidence of any residual lesion, or there is only a small area of induration, which represents the point of origin of the tumour.

The purpose of cobalt therapy is to reduce the size of the tumour to a volume suitable for single-plane interstitial curietherapy.

Second Stage: Iridium-192 Implant. The iridium implant aims to deliver a booster dose of 2000 rad in a single plane to a limited target volume in that part of the circumference of the anal canal involved ty tumour before cobalt therapy was started (Fig. 22).

The technique used at the Centre Léon Bérard was initiated by KEILING et al. (1973) in Strasbourg. The patient is admitted to hospital for preparation 1 day before implantation. General anaesthesia is preferred to an epidural block except in the case of especially frail patients with respiratory problems. The patient is put up in the lithotomy position on an operating-table, with television monitoring to check the various stages of the implantation.

Digital and endoscopic examination is performed to define the target volume and the quadrants of the anal canal into which the iridium will be implanted, and

First Protocol

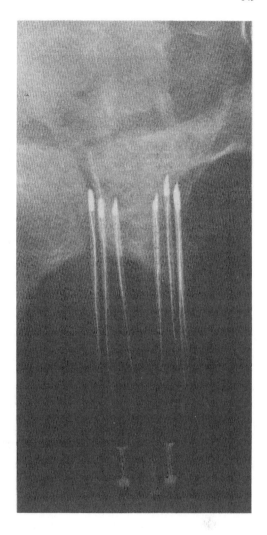

Fig. 23. X-ray film of the iridium-192 implant. Notice the good parallelism of the radioactive wires

to assess the difference in consistency and the possible residual hardening that may mark the area requiring the booster dose.

A silver grain is inserted at the lower end of the target volume, to be used as a marker visible on the TV screen and on the X-ray films to define the lowest end of the iridium wires. Great care must be taken to prevent overdosage to the anal verge, which has been irradiated with cobalt at a dose of 4200 rad. A crescent-shaped plastic template[1], 15 mm thick, with a series of holes 9 mm apart, is sutured to the peri-anal skin by four stitches. The template is placed in the quadrants of the anus originally involved by the tumour.

Steel needles 15 cm long, with their points closed by spot welding, are introduced through the holes of the template. They penetrate through the perineal

---

1 The template is built by ARPLAY Inc., IZEURE, 21110 France.

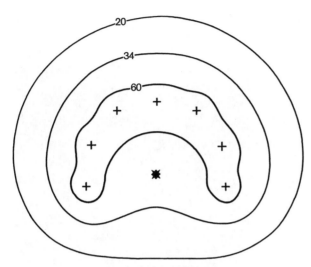

Fig. 24. Isodose distribution of the iridium-192 implant. Reference isodose distribution indicates that a dose of 60 rad/h is delivered for 1 mCi/cm

skin into the substance of the anorectal wall. They must be kept within the perirectal tissue, away from the anorectal lumen and the vaginal cavity. A finger introduced into the rectum and into the vagina will guide the penetration of the steel needles, and confirm they are positioned well. The number of steel needles depends on the extent of the tumour. Usually, five to seven steel needles are used. The length of the target volume varies from 5 cm to 7 cm, and the insertion of the neddles is carried out accordingly. An inactive lead wire, 5–7 cm long, is introduced into a needle, and the operator can check on the monitor that the steel needles are truly parallel and that they are in the right position (Fig. 23). The needles can be pushed deeper or withdrawn relative to the silver grain marker and the length of the target volume measured. Then the lead wire is withdrawn and the insertion of the iridium wires is carried out in after-loading. A last check is made on the monitor and then the ends of the steel needles containing the iridium wires are cut so that the whole implant is held in place. Preliminary dosimetry is immediately performed with a portable gamma meter, to measure the approximate dose delivered to the anal and vaginal mucosa. Then a rubber drain wrapped in soft gauze is introduced through the anus and fixed to the template. It aims at protecting the normal anorectal wall by keeping it away from the radioactive wires.

Manual dosimetry according to the "Paris system" is used to define the duration of the implantation. The dose to be given is calculated at 85% of the basal dose, which is the dose delivered at equal distance from two adjacent radioactive lines, nearest to the edge of the implant. When there are five 6 cm long wires, the dose is 60 rad/h for a linear activity of 1 mCi/cm (Fig. 24). The dose usually scheduled is 2000 rad. The lineic activity of the iridium wires used is between 2 mCi/cm and 1.3 mCi/cm. The duration of implantation varies from 18 h to 28 h. Orthogonal X-ray films are taken to check the correct positioning of the iri-

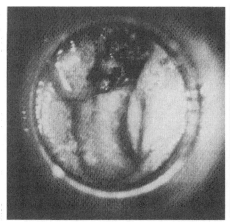 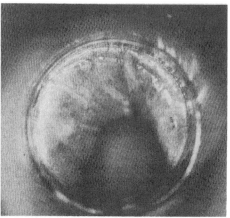

Fig. 25 a, b. Female aged 68 (obs. GAR). **a** large T^3 epidermoid carcinoma deeply infiltrating the anorectal junction and the rectovaginal wall before treatment; **b** after split-course irradiation: anal function entirely normal. Patient alive and disease-free more than 5 years after treatment

dium wires with regard to the silver grain marker and to adjust for the change of the patient's position from the lithotomy to the lying position with legs outstretched. Computerized dosimetry is corried out to define the irradiated volume.

The patients is kept strictly in a horizontal position for the duration of the application, with a low-residue diet and anticoagulation. Antibiotics are not always required.

The short duration of the curietherapy helps to make the treatment more tolerable, with short interruption of bowel activity and a low risk of thromboembolic complications.

The apparatus is removed on the ward by cutting the four stiches holding the template to the perineal skin and then withdrawing the template, steel needles, and rubber drain slowly. This procedure does not require anaesthesia because it produces very little discomfort. The patient usually leaves hospital a day later.

Tolerance. After cobalt-60 there is a slight proctitis with painful irritation of the anorectum, of the peri-anal area, and of the posterior part of the introitus, which does not last more than 2 weeks, and is easily relieved by sedative ointments. There is no radioepidermitis of the anal margin, but only a temporary erythema. Diarrhoea often occurs during the last few days of cobalt therapy and lasts 1–2 weeks, but is never a problem because the volume of bowel irradiated is very limited. One month after completion of cobalt therapy there is no more reaction, and usually the symptoms of the disease such as bleeding, feeling of bulk, discomfort in a sitting position, and trouble with defecation have completely disappeared.

The tolerance of iridium implant is usually good. In most cases, there is some pain during the treatment, which requires analgesia. The proctitis which occurs

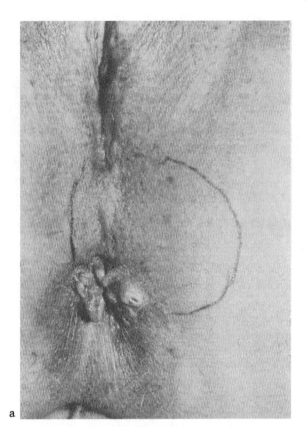

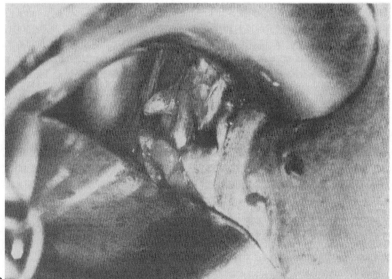

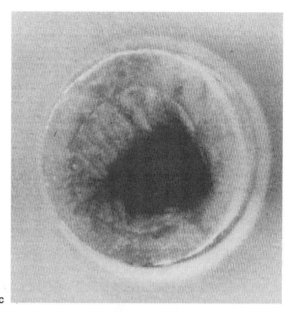

Fig. 26a–c. Female aged 74 (obs. MES). **a** T^3 epidermoid carcinoma infiltrating the perineal structures and the rectovaginal wall. The *black line* shows the extent of the tumour before treatment. **b** Endoscopic appearance of the tumour before treatment. **c** After split-course irradiation: anal function normal. Patient cured for more than 9 years

during the first few days afterwards is slight and produces mild discomfort only. The short duration of the application, which rarely exceeds 24 h, is an important factor. The pain disappears as soon as the template and the needles have been removed and a few days after returning home the patient can resume a normal active life.

In this protocol, the following points should be emphasized:
1. The moderate dosages of cobalt-60 and of iridium-192, which are distributed on a well defined target volume. The booster dose has always been applied in a single-plane implant, i.e. to a very limited area
2. The length of time (80 days) taken for the whole treatment
3. The good immediate and late tolerance by the tissues of this schedule, with a especially low rate of necrosis (5%) and no fibrosis of the peri-anal area
4. The simplicity of the protocol, which can be used for frail, elderly, and poor-risk patients
5. The effectiveness of the protocol when applied with accuracy to large T_3 tumours, which is demonstrated in Table 27.

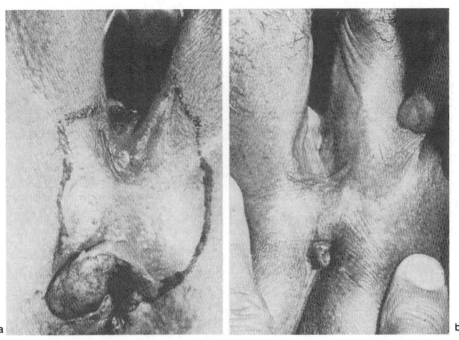

Fig. 27 a, b. Female aged 73 (obs. CHAR). Inoperable patient with severe liver cirrhosis. **a** T^4 epidermoid carcinoma of the anal canal deeply infiltrating the perineal structures with involvement of the vaginal mucosa and peri-anal area before treatment. The *black line* shows the extent of the disease. **b** After split-course irradiation, anal area and rectovaginal wall are normal: no fistula or necrosis. Patient died of liver cirrhosis free from cancer 1 year later

2. Second Protocol – Irradiation Followed by Radical Surgery

There is a group of patients whose tumours cannot be controlled by irradiation alone but require an AP excision; however, it has been shown that radical surgery by itself does not result in a high cure rate when the tumour is large and infiltrating. These patients should therefore be submitted to a pre-operative regimen that aims to reduce the size of the tumour and to destroy the microfoci situated at its periphery, with a decrease in the incidence of local and regional recurrences. This regimen should not be associated with an increase in post-operative complications.

Fig. 28. Isodose distribution of pre-operative irradiation with cobalt-60 for epidermoid carcinoma of the anal canal using two fields. Through a perineal field *(1)* a dose of 1 500 rad at 5 cm is given in five fractions. Through a sacral field *(2)* (8 × 14 cm) with 45° wedge filter a dose of 1 500 rad at 8 cm is given in five fractions. The lower end of the sacral field is 3 cm above the anal verge. The maximum dose to the anal verge is 2 200 rad. A dose of 3 000 rad is delivered to the anorectal junction and lower pararectal lymphatic drainage areas

Second Protocol

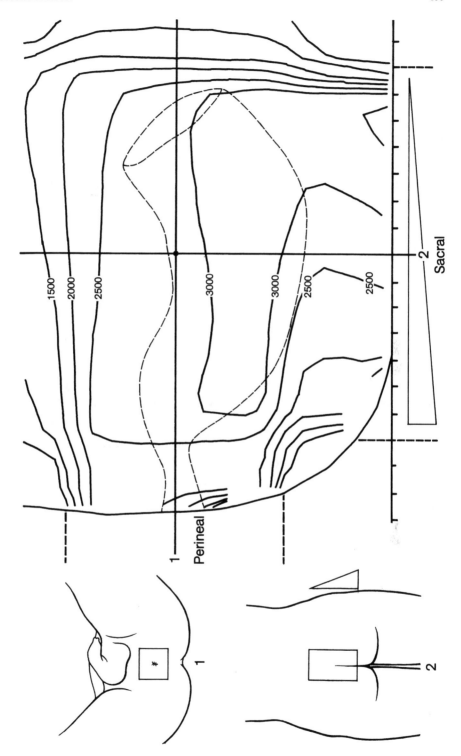

The protocol consists of delivering a dose of 3000 rad by cobalt-60 to the anal area and to the presacral area through two portals, in ten applications over 12 days (Fig. 28):
1. Through a direct perineal field 9 × 9 cm, a tumour dose of 1500 rad calculated at 5 cm depth is delivered in five fractions. The patient is irradiated in the lithotomy position, with the buttocks taped apart.
2. Through a direct sacral field 8 × 14 cm, with 45° wedge filter, a tumour dose of 1500 rad calculated at 8 cm is given in five fractions. The lower end of this field is located 3 cm above the anal verge to prevent hot spot due to overlapping of the two fields. The patient is irradiated in the prone position.

The irradiation is performed five times a week, alternating the fields every other day. The overall treatment time is 12 days. The isodose curve shown that the 3000-rad curve encompasses the whole target volume, and that the perineal skin and the anal verge receive only 2200 rad, a dose which is compatible with a normal healing of the perineal wound without delay related to the irradiation.

If 18-MeV X-rays are used, the treatment is given in 10 days and eight fractions (five on the perineal portal, three on the sacral portal) with a similar isodose curve.

Chemotherapy with 5-FU and MTC according to the protocol initiated by NIGRO et al. (1974) and NEWMAN and QUAN (1976) is usually combined with irradiation to reinforce its efficacy (see p. 140). The operation must not be carried out before the 4th week. If one takes into consideration the slow pace of shrinkage of the tumour, the best radiobiological effect is obtained between the 6th and the 8th weeks. This period is the optimal time for radical surgery. Pathological study of the operative specimens confirms the efficacy of the irradiation with some tumour-free specimens, which demonstrate the particular radiosensitivity of squamous cell carcimoma of the anal canal and of the pelvic metastatic nodes. After surgery, the healing of the perineal wound takes place with normal delay, in the same time as if pre-operative irradiation had not been performed. No complications related to radiotherapy have been observed.

3. Third Protocol – Whole-pelvic and Anal Irradiation

At the time of diagnosis, 15%–20% of anal canal carcinomas are so advanced that the lesion is unresectable. For many years in many institutions this group of patients was the only one to be referred for radiotherapy. In most cases, the irradiation has a purely palliative efficacy. However, high-dose radiation properly applied to a well-defined target volume may result in some long-term results in spite of the extent of the disease. The protocol of irradiation should be conceived in a sophisticated manner in order to give the patients the optimal results with regard to duration as well as to quality of life.

Irradiation is carried out with high-energy 18-MeV X-rays rather than cobalt. By two opposed fields a dose of 4000 rad at the mid-line is delivered to the whole pelvis over 4 weeks. The anterior field encompasses the inguinal areas but does not involve the perineum. The posterior field encompasses the anal area. This irradiation can also be carried out using three fields, one posterior and two lateral, in order to protect the bladder and small bowel and concentrate the beams on the posterior part of the pelvis. In this protocol inguinal areas are irradiated by electrons without interference with the pelvic irradiation. Booster doses up to 5500 rad are given to limited target volumes such as the anal area (by X-rays or iridium implant), pelvic mass (by X-rays), or inguinal nodes (by electrons). The overall treatment time is 6–7 weeks, with a break after the dose of 4000 rad has been distributed.

A short course of adjuvant chemotherapy (5-FU, MTC) is usually carried out during the first 5 days of irradiation, when the age and general condition of the patient do not represent a contra-indication for chemotherapy.

4. Results

Since 1971, 250 patients with squamous cell carcinoma of the anal canal have been treated according to the previously described protocols. The sex ratio was 5:1 (one male for five female patients). The average age was 65 years. One hundred and twenty-one patients have been followed up for more than 3 years. The tumours were distributed as follows:

Staging	No. of cases
T_1 or T_2	39 (32.2%)
T_3 and T_{4a}	64 (52.9%)
T_{4b}	18 (14.8%)

Limited anal canal cancers represent only one-third of the total, with large infiltrating and deeply invading tumours constituting the remainder. All the 121 patients seen between 1971 and 1978 were accepted for treatment, which consisted of radiation therapy as first approach possibly followed by surgery. This series can be divided into two subgroups: 103 resectable tumours, and 18 unresectable tumours.

The overall results are reported in Table 25. Of the 50 patients cured at 5 years, 11 had a colostomy and 40 had normal anal function. Of the 76 patients alive and well at 3 years, 16 had a colostomy and 60 had normal anal function.

Table 25. Statistics from the Centre Léon Bérard (1971–1978): Overall results

	At 5 years	At 3 years
Number of patients	85	121
Number still alive	50 (58.8%)	76 (64.6%)
Rate of death from cancer	27%	25.6%

One hundred and three patients were considered to have tumour which could have been removed by radical surgery and were followed up for more than 3 years.

a) Curative Irradiation with Cobalt-60 and Iridium-192

Ninety-seven patients had tumours which seemed to be suitable for irradiation with a curative and conservative purpose. They were treated according to the first protocol, i.e. combined irradiation by cobalt-60 and iridium-192 implant in a split-course regimen.

Sixty-six patients were followed up for more than 5 years (Table 26); 25 had T_1-T_2 tumours, 41 T_3 tumours larger than 4 cm. Forty-four (66.6%) patients were alive and well with no evidence of disease at 5 years, 36 with a normal anal function and eight with a colostomy. Surgery was performed for failure or necrosis. The 5-year survival rate was 76% for T_1-T_2 tumours and 61% for T_3. Twenty-two patients died before 5 years: 11 from cancer (16.6%), ten from intercurrent disease, and one post-operatively.

Ninety-seven patients were followed up for more than 3 years. Thirty-nine had T_1-T_2 tumours and 58 had T_3 tumours. Sixty-nine (71%) patients remained alive and well at 3 years, 56 with a normal anal function and 13 with a colostomy either for failure (eight) or for necrosis (Five). The 3-year survival rate was 79% for patients with T_1-T_2 tumours and 65.5% for patients with T_3 tumours. Size of tumours significantly influences the prognosis and the chance of preservation of anal function (Table 23).

In the group of 39 patients with T_1-T_2 tumours (4 cm or less) 31 (79%) had their tumours controlled, 29 (93%) with normal anal function, two with colostomy. In the group of 58 patients with tumours larger than 4 cm, 38 (65%) had them controlled, 27 (71%) with preservation of tha anal sphincter and 11 with colostomy.

Twenty-eight patients died: two post-operatively, 11 from intercurrent disease, 15 (15.4%) from anal cancer. In this group of 15 dead patients are included the patients who were alive at 3 years but with incurable anal lesions. The rate of death from cancer was respectively 10.2% for patients with T_1-T_2 tumours, 18.9% for patients with T_3 tumours.

It must be emphasized that the rates of death from cancer were 15.4% at 3 years and 16.6% at 5 years. One can claim that almost all patients alive and well with no evidence of disease at 3 years may be considered definitively cured.

The results obtained in this series are better than those after radical surgery with permanent colostomy. The moderate dose of radiation applied in this protocol, the fractionation, and the long overall treatment time are not only responsible for the high cure rate, the good functional results, and the low rate of severe radionecrosis, but also permit in case of failure subsequent surgery to be carried out without additional morbidity.

Local Failures. Eighteen local failures were observed, four (10.2%) with T_1-T_2 tumours, 14 (24%) with T_3 tumours. One occurred in the 4th year after irradiation;

Table 26. Results of curative irradiation of anal canal carcinoma with cobalt-60 and iridium-192[a]

	No. of cases	Alive and well	Death from cancer	Death from intercurrent disease	Post-operative death
At 5 years	66	44[b] (66.6%)	11 (16.6%)	10	1
At 3 years	97	69[c] (71%)	15 (15.4%)	11	2

[a] Centre Léon Bérard.
[b] Eight patients with colostomy.
[c] Thirteen patients with colostomy.

Table 27. Results and stage of disease following irradiation with cobalt-60 and iridium-192[a]

	Stage	No. of cases	Disease-free	Death from cancer
At 5 years	T_1-T_2	25	76%	12%
	T_3	41	61%	19.5%
At 3 years	T_1-T_2	39	31[b] (79,4%)	4 (10.2%)
	T_3	58	38[c] (65.5%)	11 (18.9%)

[a] Centre Léon Bérard.
[b] Two patients with colostomy.
[c] Eleven patients with colostomy.

all the others were observed in the 1st year. Most patients underwent radical excision; seven were cured by surgery; eight died from cancer; one died post-operatively and two from intercurrent disease, clinically free from cancer.

After conservative treatment by irradiation for squamous cell carcinoma of the anal canal, clinical assessment of the local control of the tumour is not always easy. Between the appearance and consistency of normal structures on the one hand, and neoplastic tissue or ulcerative reaction on the other hand, the difference may not be clear. Open biopsy may give rise to pain or to necrotic complications. Cytological examination of smears is extemely helpful.

Role of Cytology in Follow-up. At the Centre Léon Bérard, 52 patients with anal canal epidermoid carcinoma treated conservatively by irradiation have been followed up by cytological investigation. Malignant epidermoid cells are usually arranged in clusters with irregular outlines in poorly differentiated tumours. When differentiation and keratinization are present, neoplastic cells with nuclear abnormalities are shed singly. Blood and necrosis are also associated. Ninety-six smears were examined. Thirteen (13.6%) contained inadequate material. The relatively high rate of unsatisfactory smears is explained by the relative dryness of the anal mucosa and the absence of intestinal mucous secretion. Of the 83 evaluable smears, 54 were negative, 15 positive. In 14 other cases benign atypias were found.

Correlation between cytological and histopathological findings was studied in 17 cases. Good correlation was observed in 15 cases (88.2%): ten were negative, five were positive. One false negative result was explained by a malignant residual deposit deeply located in the anal canal structure beneath regenerated anal mucosa. One apparently false positive cytological result was observed, the biopsy being negative. However, the patient developed a local recurrence a few months later, and it was suggested that the cytology had been right, whereas biopsy had not been taken at the right place.

Pelvic Nodal Failures. Eleven patients (four with T_1-T_2 tumours, seven with T_3 tumours whose tumours were controlled locally by curative irradiation developed metastatic nodes in the mesorectum or along the pelvic wall. These nodes were discovered by palpation at follow-up examination, during the 1st year after completion of irradiation in ten cases and during the 2nd year in one case. Eight of these patients had been irradiated by perineal field only without elective irradiation of the presacral area, according to the technique used up to 1974. Only two patients irradiated by perineal and sacral fields between 1974 and 1978 developed pelvic metastatic nodes. Six patients died from cancer and one died from intercurrent disease, clinically controlled. Four are alive and well 8, 7, 5, and 3 years after treatment respectively (one patient after perineal resection, two inoperable patients after interstitial curietherapy, and one after perirectal lymphadenectomy and curietherapy).

If one considers that most failures occurred during the first 18 months and are related to a failure of primary control of the disease, the results obtained at 3 years give a strong indication of the efficacy of this type of treatment. To support this concept, there is no statistically significant difference between the rates of death from cancer at 3 and 5 years (16.6% versus 15.3%), or between the survival rates (71% and 66.6%).

To summarize *75–80% of all patients with anal canal carcinoma will have tumours suitable for treatment by the combination of cobalt-60 and iridium-192 in a split course. Two-thirds of these patients will be cured and more than three-quarters of them will have normal anal function.* Fewer than 20% of patients will die from cancer and 60% of those with T_3 tumours will be free of disease at 5 years.

b) Pre-operative Irradiation and Radical Surgery

Between 1971 and 1980, nine patients with resectable tumour not suitable for conservative treatment were treated according to the second protocol. Most lesions were either deeply infiltrating, or involved more than two-thirds of the circumference of the canal or the vaginal mucosa, or were associated with pelvic metastatic nodes. They were resectable and the patients were fit for surgery. In all cases the irradiation resulted in relief of symptoms such as tenesmus and pain, and in s substantial reduction in the size of the lesions. Abdominoperineal resection was performed between the 4th and 8th weeks following completion of the irradiation. The operative specimen showed no more tumour in three cases. In the six other cases, the lesion was considered histologically active. After operation there were no additional complications related to the pre-operative irradiation and the perineal wounds healed within the usual time. Among the six pa-

Table 28. Results of treatment for anal canal carcinoma: Resectable tumours[a]

	No. of cases	Alive and well	No colostomy	Death from cancer
At 5 years	72	47[b] (65%)	36 (50%)	18%
At 3 years	103	72[b] (70%)	56 (54%)	17.5%

[a] Centre Léon Bérard.
[b] Seventy-five percent of the patients controlled had no colostomy.

tients followed up for over 3 years, three are alive and well, disease-free, one after 6 years, two after more than 3 years; two patients treated who were found to have metastatic nodes in the operative specimen died 6 and 8 years later of pelvic recurrences; one died from intercurrent disease. It must be emphasized that all patients treated according to the first or second protocol had resectable tumours which could have been treated by radical surgery, and results obtained by irradiation with or without subsequent surgery (Table 28) can be compared with those of surgery alone.

c) Whole-pelvic Irradiation for Unresectable Tumours

Eighteen patients submitted to whole-pelvic irradiation for unresectable tumour had huge, fixed tumours with invasion of the surrounding structures. In three cases the anus was so narrowed that a colostomy was needed before any other treatment. Many lesions had widely involved the perineal area and in most cases there were not only inguinal metastatic nodes, but also pelvic masses more or less fixed to the pelvic wall. One patient had a lung metastasis and a left supraclavicular node. The irradiation was always well tolerated, and the general condition of the patient was often improved by the relief of the pain and discomfort. The remission varied from short periods to more than 2 years. Two patients died from intercurrent disease and the post-mortem examination showed no tumour.

Of the 18 patients followed up for over 3 years, four patients are alive and well, disease-free, after 9, 8, 6 and 3 years respectively. All of them had large lesions with extensive lymphatic spread throughout the pelvis. The disappearance of these lesions after treatment showed a high degree of radiosensitivity, and suggests that radiation therapy should be applied at high dosage with an appropriate fractionation for advanced anal canal cancers with agressive intent. The data demonstrate that some tumours apparently incurable because of their extent are more radiosensitive than they were thought to be and can sometimes be controlled.

Comparison of Results. Table 29 summarizes the results obtained by using the three protocols. These results demonstrate that radiation therapy as first approach must be the rule in the treatment of almost all patients with squamous cell carcinoma of the anal canal.

Table 29. Epidermoid carcinoma of the anal canal: Results according to resectability of tumour[a]

	No. of cases	Alive and well at more than 5 years	Tumours controlled without colostomy
Resectable tumours	72	47	36
Unresectable tumours	13	3	3
	85	50 (58.8%)	39 (78%)

[a] Centre Léon Bérard.

"The series updated in February 1982 showed the following results: In the group of resectable tumours, in 81 patients followed up for more than 5 years, the rate of survival NED was 64%. In 113 patients followed up for more than 3 years, the rate of survival NED was 67%. The rate of death from cancer was the same at 5 and 3 years: 18,5%. Among the patients clinically controlled, the rates for patients cured without colostomy were respectively 86% and 77%.

In the group of unresectable tumours, of 16 patients followed up for more than 5 years, three were alive and well. Of 24 patients followed up for more than 3 years, four had tumor clinically controlled."

5. Lymphatic Spread

Lymph node involvement is common in patients with epidermoid carcinoma of the anal canal. In the present series, 54 patients (44.6%) developed regional metastases which were located in the inguinal or/and pelvic area.

a) Inguinal Metastasis

The incidence of inguinal spread according to the literature is 20%–25%. Of the 121 patients treated between 1971 and 1978 and followed up for more than 3 years, 28 (23%) developed groin metastases. The malignant nature of the lymph nodes was demonstrated in the operative specimens or by aspiration biopsy. Involvement of the inguinal lymph nodes was more common in infiltrating tumours larger than 4 cm in diameter – 22 cases (27%) – than in limited carcinomas of the anal canal – six cases (15%).

In 14 cases inguinal node involvement was present at the time of diagnosis of the anal tumours (synchronous metastases). In 14 cases, inguinal node metastases occurred during the follow-up period (metachronous metastases). It has already been emphasized that the presence of groin metastasis before treatment of the primary tumours has a poor prognostic significance. The series from the Centre Léon Bérard conforms to this rule. Of the 14 patients with synchronous groin metastasis, nine (64%) died of cancer, whereas three are alive and well between 3 and 9 years later and two died of intercurrent disease clinically controlled. In the group of patients with synchronous metastasis, 12 patients had T_3 and T_4 tumours, whereas two had limited anal canal cancer. Both these patients have had their disease controlled for longer than 6 and 10 years respectively. In 14 patients, inguinal metastases occurred after treatment of the primary tumour, the inguinal clinical examination being negative at the time of pre-treatment evaluation. In nine patients, the groin metastases were discovered during the first 3 months. In three cases inguinal metastases occurred later. Five patients died of cancer, nine (64%) were alive and well clinically cured. These figures are rather similar to those reported by GOLDEN and HORSLEY (1976).

The prognosis remains favourable even when early metachronous groin metastases occur, although these metastases must have been present as subclinical disease at the time of presentation.

The treatment of inguinal metastatic lymph nodes consisted of superficial or limited block dissection in most cases. One patient underwent a radical groin dissection. In all cases post-operative irradiation at a dose of 4500 rad over 5–6 weeks was carried out, generally with cobalt-60 (3000 rad) and electrons (1500 rad).

In ten patients, definitive irradiation of the groin was performed because of their poor general condition or because of the extent of the anal tumour; needle biopsy had always confirmed the lymph node involvement by a squamous cell carcinoma. Of this group of ten patients three remained alive and well, disease-free, after 10, 5 and 3½ years. One had a local excision of a residual nodule in the groin, which proved to be tumour-free, and died from intercurrent disease in the 4th year without recurrence.

It is not widely accepted that irradiation of inguinal metastatic nodes related to epidermoid carcinoma is an effective treatment. Two patients not included in the series with clinically and cytologically involved inguinal nodes were treated more recently by pre-operative irradiation followed 5 weeks later by limited groin dissection. In neither was there any tumour in the excised lymph nodes.

These results show that inguinal nodes involved by an epidermoid carcinoma originating in the anal canal are very radiosensitive, and that irradiation may play a major role either post-operatively or as a primary definitive procedure.

Tolerance of inguinal irradiation is good, provided the technique is accurate and the dose reasonable. There is no sclerosis of the groin and no oedema of the leg. As a rule a combination of cobalt-60 and electrons is advisable. Complications were observed in two cases, after incorrect technique (high-dose irradiation with cobalt-60 only). They consisted of fractures of the iliopubic bone or the hip. One was treated medically with a satisfactory result. The other underwent prosthesis. It must be borne in mind that high-dose radiation applied to the hip may produce trophic changes in bones in elderly patients. This complication is readily prevented by using electron therapy for one-third of the dose distributed to the groins. The results are shown in Table 30.

This series confirms the bad prognostic significance of early lymphatic dissemination to the groin and the good chance of cure after proper treatment if the lymphatic spread is detected during the follow-up period. The results emphasize the place which should be given to radiation therapy used post-operatively or on

Table 30. Inguinal lymph node involvement: Results after treatment in 121 cases (1971–1978)[a]

	No. of cases	Alive and well more than 3 years disease-free	Deaths from cancer	Deaths from interc. dis.
Synchronous groin metastasis	14	3 (21.9%)	9 (64%)	2
Metachronous groin metastasis	14	9 (64%)	5 (35%)	0
	28 (23%)	12 (42.8%)	14 (50%)	

[a] Centre Léon Bérard.

Table 31. Pelvic metastatic nodes[a]

		No. of cases
Nature	Lymph nodes	36
	Venous node of permeation (or in-transit metastasis)	2
Location	Perirectal (haemorrhoidal)	34
	Along the pelvic wall	4
Site of anal tumour	Above the dentate line	35
	Below the dentate line	3
Time of discovery	Synchronous	22
	Metachronous	16

[a] Centre Léon Bérard.

its own in the treatment of the inguinal metastatic nodes. It is advisable not to perform prophylactic groin dissection of the inguinal areas when the patient can be carefully followed up.

b) Pelvic Node Metastasis

In the series of 121 patients with carcinoma of the anal canal seen at the Centre Léon Bérard between 1971 and 1978, pelvic node metastases were found in 38 cases (31.4%), either in operative specimens (two) or by rectal digital examination (36). The malignant nature of the nodes was proved by histology or cytology in 18 cases, and assumed on clinical grounds in 20 cases because of the extension of the pelvic mass and the fatal course of the disease, or because of the favourable response to irradiation. The shrinkage and the disappearance of the metastatic nodules after high-dose radiotherapy has demonstrated that pelvic nodes have the same radiosensitivity as the primary tumour. Some operative specimens have shown that malignant deposits in pelvic nodes could be entirely destroyed by radiation therapy. The general features of the pelvic nodes are reported in Table 31. The lymphatic origin of the pelvic nodes was assumed in all except two cases, where operative specimens showed that they were in-transit metastases or venous nodes of permeation.

Female aged 72: Pain in the anal area for 6 months considered to be related to constipation and haemorrhoids. Large squamous cell carcinoma of the anal canal, 6 cm long, very infiltrating, having

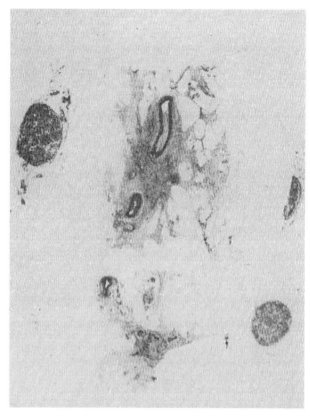

Fig. 29. Obs. BRAI. Operative specimen from AP resection: venous node of permeation or in-transit metastasis discovered at rectal digital examination in a patient with T^3 epidermoid carcinoma of the anal canal. Two normal lymph nodes are visible

invaded three-quarters of the circumference and narrowing the anal orifice. Rectal digital examination was painful.

Cobalt therapy by perineal field was started but re-examination under general anaesthesia was performed a few days later when a tumour dose of 1500 rad had been delivered. Rectal digital examination showed a hard nodule, 1.5 cm in diameter, located 4 cm above the primary tumour in the mesorectum. The patient underwent an AP resection 3 weeks later. The nodule had substantially shrunk. Pathological investigation of the operative specimen showed that the nodule was not a metastatic lymph node but a venous node of permeation developed in a vasculonervous pedicle (Fig. 29). The patient recovered from the operation but died 10 month later from a second primary adenocarcinoma of the stomach (obs. BRAI).

Most pelvic nodes were located in the mesorectum and seemed to be attached to the lateral or posterior part of the rectal wall. However, in four cases the nodules were located anteriorly either in the rectovaginal wall (three) or fixed to the prostate (one). In seven cases the nodes were situated along the pelvic wall (hypogastric lymphatic chain).

The distance between the anal tumour and the nodes varies from 2 cm to 7 cm. The average size of the nodes was 2 cm in diameter. They were usually big-

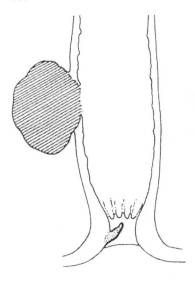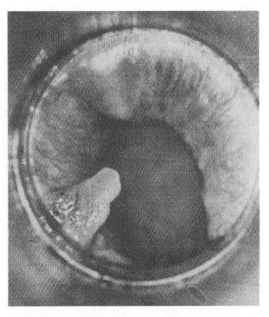

Fig. 30. Obs. CAL. Big pararectal metastatic lymph node ulcerated in the rectal wall secondary to a small spike-shaped epidermoid carcinoma located below the dentate line. An AP resection after preoperative irradiation showed no active tumour cells in the anus or in the metastatic lymph node. Patient alive and well more than 3 years after treatment

ger that those found in case of rectal adenocarcinoma. In 12 cases there was a tethered or fixed mass larger than 3 cm.

Although metastatic nodes in the pelvis are more common in advanced cancers, they can be seen in small lesions less than 4 cm in diameter (Figs. 30 and 31). In the great majority of cases (46) the tumour was located in the upper part of the anal canal; in three cases the lesion was located entirely below the dentate line. These findings illustrate the necessity of including under the heading of anal canal cancers these tumours located in the lower part of the canal.

According to the time of discovery of pelvic metastases, one can distinguish between synchronous (22) and metachronous (16) cases.

Pelvic nodes were present at the time of diagnosis of the anal canal tumour in 22 cases, and in one case a pelvic mass was discovered at a routine examination, proved on biopsy to be a metastasis of a squamous cell carcinoma, and led to discovery of a small carcinoma of the anal canal, which was asymptomatic (see first case below).

Female aged 58: Before operation for gallstones a routine rectal digital examination discovered a big mass in the pelvis in the left pararectal area. The mass was 6 cm in diameter, tethered, with ulceration of the rectal mucosa. A biopsy proved that it was a lymph node involved by a squamous cell carcinoma. No symptom in the anal area. Anoscopy showed a small, elevated spike-shaped lesion 1.5 cm long, 4 mm in diameter, implanted in the lowest part of the anal canal below the dentate line on the left side. Biopsy: squamous cell carcinoma (Fig. 30). Irradiation by 18-MeV photons at a dose of 4000 rad over 4 weeks. Disappearance of the anal lesion. Moderate shrinkage of the pelvic mass, which had become more mobile. Four months later, an AP resection was performed. Operative speci-

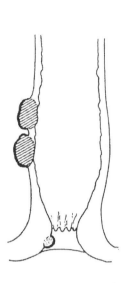 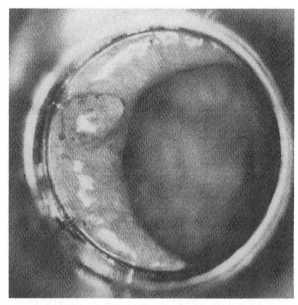

Fig. 31. Obs. SCI. Small button-like squamous cell carcinoma of the lower anal canal associated with two pararectal metastatic lymph nodes. After split-course irradiation with cobalt-60 and iridium implant, a perirectal lymphadenectomy showed no active tumour. Control of the disease for more than 3 years after treatment

men showed that there was no active tumour but only keratinized plaques representing the original tumour in the lymph node. Patient alive and well 3 years later (obs. CAL) (Fig. 30).

In the next case the first sign of the disease was a sciatic pain due to a significant pelvic adenopathy, which preceded the discovery of the anal canal tumour by 6 months.

Female aged 42: For 6 months left sciatic pain not relieved by medical treatment. For 3 months tenderness of the anal region. Discovery of a large infiltrating squamous cell carcinoma of the anal canal astride the dentate line, involving the lowest part of the rectum on the left side. Rectal digital examination showed a big mass 4 cm in diameter fixed to the left pelvic wall 10 cm above the anal verge. Irradiation by photons 18-MeV doses): 4500 rad to the anal canal and 4000 rad to the posterior pelvic area plus 1000 rad boost to the left pelvic node, resulted in a relief of the sciatic pain and disappearance of the lesions. Alive with palliative treatment after 30 months (obs. YVA).

The following case is an example of synchronous metastatic node histologically controlled by irradiation.

Female aged 56: A few weeks after a little rectal bleeding, a very small button-like tumour of the lower part of the anal canal below the dentate line was observed. Histology: squamous cell carcinoma. Rectal digital examination found two pararectal metastatic nodes: the first 3 cm in diameter, 7 cm above the anal verge; the second 2 cm higher, 2.5 cm in diameter. Aspiration biopsy of the first node: squamous cell carcinoma. No other sign of dissemination. CEA normal (Fig. 31). Irradiation with photons 18 MeV, dose 4000 rad, to the posterior part of the pelvis and anus plus booster dose of 1000 rad to the nodes. Two months later, disappearance of the anal lesion and of the metastatic nodes. Iridium implant of the anal area and of the pararectal space in the area where the nodes had been found. Two months later, mesenteric and perirectal lymphadenectomy. Operative specimen cancer-free. Patient alive and well with normal anal function 3 years later (obs. SCI) (Fig. 31).

Table 32. Incidence of pelvic recurrences after control of the anal tumour by irradiation according to technique employed[a]

Period of time and target volume	No. of cases locally controlled	Rate of pelvic recurrence
1971–1974 Irradiation confined to the anal area	37	9 (24.3%)
1974–1978 Irradiation extended to presacral area	30	2 (6.6%)

[a] Centre Léon Bérard.

These data demonstrate the usefulness of the search for the pelvic nodes at the time of the pre-treatment evaluation. Among the 22 patients with synchronous pelvic metastatic nodes, 11 died from cancer; one died from intercurrent disease, locally controlled, and ten (45%) were alive and well 3–10 years, later six of them having had an AP resection after pre-operative irradiation. Four operative specimens were free from active tumour-cells: the neoplastic tissue had been entirely destroyed by radiotherapy. Two had active tumour-cells in the nodes. Four patients had been treated by irradiation only and had normal anal function.

Metachronous pelvic metastasis was observed in 16 cases. Five were associated with local relapse of the primary tumour, whereas in 11 patients they occurred after local control of the anal tumour. Of the five patients with local and nodal recurrences, four died of cancer and one died of intercurrent disease. The series of 11 patients with pelvic nodal metastases only must be divided into two subgroups according to the technique of irradiation:
1. Of the 37 patients treated by irradiation confined to the anal area between 1971 and 1974 whose tumours were locally controlled, nine developed pelvic nodal recurrences.
2. Of the 30 patients treated by irradiation extended to the presacral area between 1974 and 1978 whose tumours were locally controlled, two developed pelvic nodal recurrences.

The comparison of the incidence of pelvic nodal recurrences in the two groups of patients followed up for over 3 years has borderline statistical significance. This difference is not due to the selection of patients treated during the second period compared with the first period. On the contrary, the percentage of T_3 tumours was higher in the second period. Neither is it due to the length of the follow-up period, since most pelvic recurrences occurred during the first 2 years. It is related to the prophylactic effectiveness of irradiation against subclinical pelvic metastasis of the perirectal area (Table 32).

To summarize, one can state that prophylactic irradiation of the posterior pelvic and presacral areas at the time of treatment of anal canal lesion has proved to be efficient in decreasing the incidence of pelvic failures.

Of the 11 patients with anal tumours, controlled who developed pelvic node recurrences, five died from cancer; six are alive and well, two after AP resection, one after perirectal lymphadenectomy (see below), and three after irradiation only.

Female aged 64: Small, poorly differentiated squamous cell carcinoma of the lowest part of the anal canal, below the dentate line on the right side. Curative irradiation by cobalt-60 to the perineal

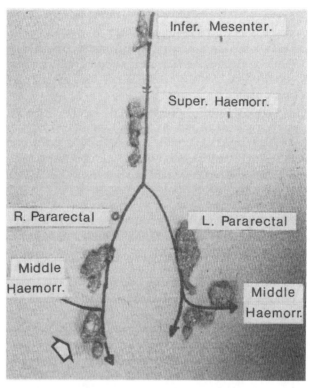

Fig. 32. Obs. BRES. Operative specimen of a mesenteric and perirectal lymphadenectomy for a patient treated by split-course irradiation for a carcinoma of the anal canal that was locally controlled, who developed a pararectal metastatic node discovered at follow-up examination. The metastatic lymph node is indicated by the *arrow on the right side*. There was only one lymph node involved. The other lymph nodes removed were negative. Patient alive and well 3 years after treatment

and presacral area according to the first protocol. Two months later, iridium-192 interstitial implant with five wires 5 cm long. Dose: 2000 rad. Seven months later, the follow-up examination showed a pararectal nodule 1½ cm in diameter, hard, mobile, located on the right side, considered to be an involved lymph node. The patient underwent a mesenteric and perirectal lymphadenectomy which demonstrated that the node palpated was a lymph node of the haemorrhoidal chain involved by an epidermoid carcinoma more differentiated than the primary tumour. The node was easily removed without resection of the bowel. No other node was involved. One month later an iridium interstitial implant with two wires directed to the rectal wall at the place of the metastatic node was carried out. Dose: 3000 rad. Patient alive and well, cancer-free, 3 years later (obs. BRES) (Fig. 32).

It must be added that in two patients a small hard nodule in the rectovaginal wall was discovered 6 months after curative irradiation of a tumour of the anal canal. Biopsy showed that it was a benign, fibrotic nodule.

Of the 38 patients with pelvic node metastasis, either synchronous or metachronous, followed up for more than 3 years: 20 (53%) died from cancer; 2 died from intercurrent disease with no evidence of cancer; and 16 (42%) were alive and well, disease-free, most of them more than 5 years after treatment. Eight of the 16 had a colostomy, eight had normal anal function. Of the 121 patients treat-

ed between 1971 and 1978, twelve (10%) had simultaneous or successive involvement of pelvic and inguinal lymph nodes. Only two had their tumours controlled; 11 died from cancer. Involvement of both routes of lymphatic spread has a poor prognostic significance. In conclusion, our experience shows that:
1. Pelvic nodal metastases can be detected by careful digital examination. Systematic search for lymphatic spread is required at the pre-treatment evaluation as well as during the follow-up period of patients with cancer of the anal canal, whatever the size and the site of tumour.
2. Radical surgery is not the only approach to the management of pelvic nodes. In many instances, and especially in poor-risk patients, radiation therapy for pelvic nodes has proved to be efficient. In all cases of pelvic spread, irradiation should be used either in association with an operative procedure, or on its own.
3. The rate of control of pelvic nodes by surgery and/or radiotherapy is about 40%. The prognosis of lymphatic spread into the pelvis is not as bad as expected, even when there is pelvic dissemination at the time of the diagnosis of carcinoma of the anal canal.
4. In the absence of palpable nodes in the pelvis at the pre-treatment investigation, prophylactic irradiation of pelvic drainage areas is justified in all patients.

To summarize, it can be stated that involvement of lymph nodes, whether pelvic or inguinal, is extremely common, since it is observed in nearly one in two patients with carcinoma of the anal canal. In all cases this problem must be considered in the therapeutic approach.

XIV. Indications for Treatment

1. Management of Tumours of the Anal Canal

Important progress has been made in our knowledge of the radiation response of squamous cell carcinoma of the anal canal, with a substantial improvement in local control and preservation of anal function. The respective roles of radiotherapy and surgery are not the same as they were 10 years ago. With the exception of the rare anal cancer complicated by major sepsis, radical surgery is no longer the first approach to the management of anal canal squamous cell carcinoma.

a) Small Cancer Treated by Local Excision

Local excision should only be regarded as an excisional biopsy, not as a definitive treatment of anal canal cancer, because of the incidence of recurrences. In all cases, even if the pathologist who studies the operative specimen considers that the removal has been complete, post-operative irradiation must be carried out with cobalt-60 and iridium-192 in a split course. This irradiation aims at preventing not only local but also nodal failures.

It is known that early cancer of the canal, even located below the dentate line and theoretically amenable to local excision, may give rise to pelvic nodal spread, and irradiation of the presacral area is always necessary. The irradiation may be started 2 or 3 weeks after local excision and is well tolerated.

b) Cobalt-60 and Iridium-192 in a Split Course

Most tumours are suitable for such an approach, which has proved to be very reliable for T_1, T_2, and T_3 lesions, which represent about 80% of cases. This protocol aims to control the tumour with the preservation of anal function. It can be applied irrespective of the age and general condition of the patient, or of the histological type of the tumour, squamous, basaloid or cloacogenic.

Adjuvant chemotherapy with 5 FU and MTC during the first 5 days of irradiation can also be used, especially for T_3 tumours, when the general condition of the patient is satisfactory.

c) Pre-operative Irradiation and Radical Surgery

Some tumours are resectable but not suitable for a curative irradiation with preservation of the anal function. When such cancers are encountered in healthy patients, they can be treated by radical surgery, but the chances of cure are improved after combined radiotherapy and surgery.
This group comprises:
1. T_{4a} tumours with invasion of the vaginal mucosa
2. T_3 tumours with palpable metastatic nodes in the mesorectum
3. Deeply infiltrating and annular tumours which involve the entire circumference of the sphincter muscle or more than ⅔ of the circumference
4. Muco-epidermoid carcinomas.

In such cases, a combined approach consisting of irradiation for 12 days and chemotherapy with 5-FU and MTC for the first 5 days, followed by AP resection 6–8 weeks later, gives patients the best chance of cure.

d) Treatment of Unresectable Tumours

One group of patients have large tumours that infiltrate the neighbouring structures extensively, with or without pelvic metastatic nodes. The tumours are fixed and the involved area is so large that the tumour is not considered amenable to radical surgery. Sometimes colostomy is required before any other treatment because of the degree of stenosis of the anal canal. These advanced cancers are only suitable for irradiation, preferably combined with adjuvant chemotherapy. Irradiation usually relieves pain, tenesmus, discharge, and bleeding for a period, which varies according to the extent of disease and its radiosensitivity.

The long-term results are poor, but in some cases there are surprising successes which justify careful planning of aggressive treatment.

In these protocols radical surgery has no place as first approach in the management of epidermoid carcinoma of the anal canal. In the great majority of cases irradiation and adjuvant chemotherapy are given for all purposes. If radical irradiation fails or necrosis occurs, major surgery is needed and may be carried out with a good prospect of control of the disease in most cases.

2. Management of Lymph Node Metastasis

a) Inguinal Lymph Nodes

In most published series, the treatment of inguinal metastatic lymph nodes is exclusively surgical; the role of radiation therapy is reduced to a palliative purpose applied to inoperable metastatic glands. One can state that the place of irradiation should be re-evaluated, with close cooperation between surgeons and radiotherapists.

Surgery

Therapeutic Groin Dissection. GOLIGHER (1975) has described two variants of operation: a superficial inguinal gland dissection without dividing the inguinal ligament and entering the pelvis; a more radical dissection, which involves division of the inguinal ligament and removal of the glands along the external and common illiac vessels, as well as the superficial inguinal nodes

Both of these operations are known to have a post-operative period often troubled by a considerable morbidity, with discharge of lymph, lymphatic collection in the groin, necrosis of the skin flaps, and lymphoedema of the leg, which may seriously prolong the process of convalescence.

HOLMES et al. (1977), studying the surgical management of melanoma, defined technical procedures that aim to reduce the post-operative morbidity of groin dissection. These guidelines are applicable to patients with carcinoma of the anal canal.

The skin incision which is placed in the inguinal crease is curved towards the anterior superior iliac spine. The inferior skin flaps are raised only to the extent that is necessary to dissect the contents of the femoral triangle. This dissection includes the subcutaneous fat and lymphatic tissue down to the adventitia of the femoral vessels. The inferior extent of the dissection terminates at the point where the sartorius muscle crosses the adductor. Extending the dissection larger does contribute to rendering the inferior flap ischemic. The upper flap is elevated to the level of the anterior superior iliac spine laterally and medially one half the distance from the pubic tubercle to the umbilicus. The fat between Camper's fascia and the external oblique aponeurosis is reflected inferiorly to meet the specimen from the femoral triangle of Poupart's ligament. The inguinal ligament is elevated and the highest inguinal node, Cloquet's node, is removed. The specimen is carefully dissected by the pathologist and any suspicious lymph nodes are examined by frozen section.

If no positive lymph nodes are found by frozen section the operation is then completed without an iliac obturator node dissection. However, if positive inguinal nodes are found on frozen section, an iliac obturator dissection is performed. This retroperitoneal node dissection is performed without an additional skin incision. The inguinal ligament is not divided: the sartorius muscle is detached from its origin from the anterior superior iliac spine and sutured to the inguinal ligament over the femoral vessels. After this has been accomplished suction catheters are inserted superiorly above, not through the upper flap.

This procedure is commonly used at the Centre Léon Bérard. However, in very elderly patients or in patients in poor general condition, instead of inguinal block dissection, a limited dissection consisting of removal of the glands obviously involved may be carried out, as long as post-operative irradiation is performed a few days later. The rationale of such an operation is based both on the pathological findings, which show that in most cases only a few nodes are involved, and on the fact that radiation therapy for inguinal metastatic nodes has proved to be more efficient than it is usually thought to be. After such limited operations there are few complications and no delay in wound healing.

Prophylactic Dissection. The value of prophylactic groin dissection in the curative treatment of carcinoma of the anal canal with no clinically involved glands has been subject to controversy. PACK and REKERS (1942) advocated bilateral groin dissection performed at the time of the resection of the primary tumour or a few weeks later. In contrast, STEARNS and QUAN (1970) have demonstrated the futility of doing prophylactic inguinal node dissection. In the series of the Memorial Hospital, he showed that 53 bilateral operations would have to be done for the doubtful salvage of three patients, and that this operation was associated with considerable morbidity. WOLFE (1968) and BEAHRS (1979) have the same opinion. GOLIGHER (1975) considers that most operative complications "outweigh the possible gain of prophylactic dissection", provided a careful follow-up can be performed with patients instructed of the necessity for systematic examination, and that inguinal node dissection should be reserved for use when the nodes become involved. GOLIGHER (1975) applied this rule except in three patients, who were not able to guarantee regular follow-up attendances, and for whom he advised prophylactic block dissection, with the removal of positive glands in one patient.

It may seem inconsistent to carry out a prophylactic treatment of pelvic nodes by surgery or radiotherapy, while the inguinal area remains untreated. Inguinal nodes can be readily observed and dissected at the first sign of involvement, whereas pelvic nodal spread, even if some lymph nodes are within reach of the examining finger, cannot be assessed with the same accuracy.

Radiation Therapy. Irradiation of the inguinal metastatic nodes may be applied in three ways: as post-operative treatment, definitive or palliative treatment, or prophylactic treatment when lymph nodes in the other groin are involved. The objective is to deliver a depth dose of 4500–5500 rad to a target volume including the inguinocrural area and the retrocrural area, without giving rise to complications such as sclerosis of the groin and lymphoedema of the leg.

The technique involves a combination of gamma rays of cobalt-60 and 13-MeV electrons. Usually, in the case of post-operative or prophylactic irradiation, a dose of 3000 rad of cobalt-60 calculated at 4 cm depth is given over 3 weeks. Then a booster dose of 1500 rad of electrons is given over 1½ weeks. The overall treatment time is 4½ weeks. For definitive or palliative treatment a total dose of 5500 rad is given in a split course. Firstly, a dose of 4000 rad is given over 4 weeks. Then a break of 3 weeks takes place and a booster dose of 1500 rad is given on a reduced portal, taking advantage of the shrinkage of the metastatic mass. The overall treatment time is 8½ weeks. Such treatment is well tolerated and there are no major sequelae.

Post-operative Irradiation. After groin dissection the previously scheduled irradiation should be started as early as possible after surgery, usually in the 3rd post-operative week. That means that the inguinal scar heals quite quickly, without lasting lymphorrhea or necrosis of skin flaps. The surgeon should be aware of this point, and should not carry out a very extensive groin dissection to prevent post-operative morbidity.

Definitive or Palliative Irradiation. When groin dissection is contra indicated because of the presence of inoperable metastatic nodes, or because of the extent of the anal canal tumour, which is considered to be unresectable or inoperable, all chances of partial or complete remission, or in some cases of long-term survival, rely on the radiation therapy. After needle biopsy of the inguinal nodes the irradiation is conducted at the appropriate dose on a target volume adapted to the extent of the disease in the pelvis and in the groin. In such cases, lymphangiography is helpful in defining the extent of lymphatic spread and the target volume.

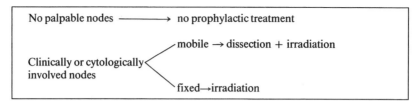

Fig. 33. Treatment of inguinal node metastasis

Prophylactic Groin Irradiation. ROUSSEAU et al. (1973), of the Institut Curie, has used irradiation as a prophylactic procedure for clinically univolved inguinal areas at the same time as the treatment of the anal tumour. He recorded three subsequent metastatic inguinal nodes in a series of 128 cases. Prophylactic irradiation may be justified after unilateral groin dissection for metastatic nodes. In such cases the irradiation is applied simultaneously to the dissected groin as a post-operative measure and to the other groin as a prophylactic measure. This protocol applied at the Centre Léon Bérard has proved to be efficient. In a series of 47 cases, no recurrence was observed in the prophylactically irradiated inguinal area. Groin irradiation may also be justified in the case of pelvic metastatic nodes with clinically uninvolved inguinal glands. The general rules of management of metastasis to the groin are summarized by the flow-diagram in Fig. 33.

Close collaboration between surgeon and radiotherapist is required in the management of groin metastasis, because the respective roles of surgery and radiation therapy should be discussed in each individual case.

b) Pelvic Lymph Nodes

Pelvic lymphatic spread represents one of the main arguments in favour of radical excision, whether combined or not with iliac lymphadenectomy for carcinoma of the anal canal. In the absence of palpable nodes, the incidence of potential pelvic spread is a justification of treatment whatever the size and the site of the tumour of the anal canal. It has been demonstrated that early and limited anal cancer may give rise to pararectal metastatic nodes, even when the tumour originates below the dentate line. In the past, AP resection was considered to be the only reliable procedure for treatment of actual and potential pelvic spread. Now, however, with modern improvements in technical approach, radiation therapy has demonstrated its effectiveness as an additional or a primary therapy of nodal extension to the pelvis.

Several presentations may be encountered. The treatment may be either prophylactic, in the absence of palpable pelvic metastatic nodes, or directed to palpable masses which may or may not be resectable. The anal lesion may be operable or inoperable according to the extent of the disease. Lastly, the treatment can be conceived as part of the therapy for the primary anal tumour, or directed to pelvic recurrence after control of the anal lesion by radical or conservative procedures. Surgical procedures consist of: (a) AP resection with or without iliac

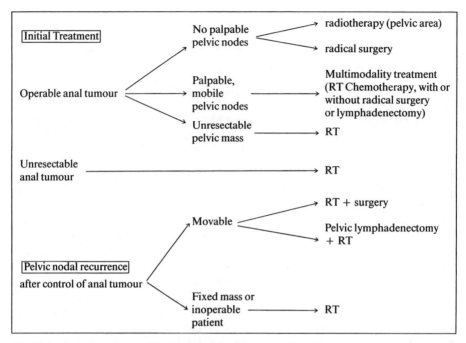

Fig. 34. Anal canal carcinoma: Management of pelvic metastatic nodes

lymphadenectomy, and (b) mesenteric and perirectal lymphadenectomy (described on p. 47). Radiation therapy consists of external irradiation with cobalt-60 or high-energy photons, possibly combined with iridium-192 implant for low-lying pararectal nodes. The principles of management are given in the flow-diagram in Fig. 34.

Initial Treatment. When anal tumour is suitable for curative and conservative treatment, in the absence of palpable pelvic metastatic lymph nodes, the irradiation is applied to anal and presacral areas according to the first protocol. In case of pelvic node metastasis not larger than 3 cm, irradiation can be used with a booster dose to the involved lymph node. If the regression of the lymphatic mass and anal tumour is satisfactory, a conservative procedure may be used as long as a mesenteric and perirectal lymphadenectomy is performed 2 months later. When the tumour or the metastatic node does not disappear completely, then radical surgery is essential. Radiotherapy is the only procedure used in the case of unresectable anal tumour or fixed pelvic node metastasis.

Pelvic Nodal Recurrence During the Follow-up Period. After control of the primary tumour by a conservative procedure such as well-planned irradiation, the discovery of a metastatic lymph node in the mesorectum leads to surgery, either conservative (mesenteric and perirectal lymphadenectomy combined with postoperative irradiation), or radical, i.e. AP resection possibly combined with pre-operative irradiation. When the pelvic mass is fixed to the pelvic wall or when the patient is inoperable, high-dose irradiation is concentrated to the involved area, but the result of treatment is usually palliative.

The application of these guidelines and the substantial role of radiation therapy in the management of pelvic spread are justified by long-term results obtained by a more aggressive, though not always radical, approach to this problem.

XV. Epidermoid Carcinoma of the Anal Margin

1. General Features

Carcinoma of the anal margin arises from the peri-anal skin outside the anal verge, and is often considered to behave like epidermoid cancer elsewhere in the skin. This is true, but it would be wrong to treat peri-anal carcinoma like any other skin cancer, because carcinoma of the anal margin is in the immediate vicinity of the anal orifice, in a region which is in direct continuity with the modified skin of the lower anal canal. In addition, the underlying perineal soft tissues do not tolerate high-dose radiation very well. Moreover, buttocks and peri-anal are a support a substantial part of the body weight in the sitting position, and any abnormality in this area may cause serious discomfort for the patient.

The peri-anal region is drained by efferent collecting lymphatic trunks, which run forwards and outwards in the fatty cellular subcutaneous tissue of the perineum and genitocrural fold, to terminate in the medial group of superficial inguinal lymph nodes. The peri-anal region does not drain into the mesenteric nodes. Tumours arising from the anal margin are usually well-differentiated squamous cell carcinomas (prickle-cell-type tumours), producing abundant keratin, and often show only superficial invasion. They can metastasize to the inguinal nodes and to the iliac nodes. This type of epithelioma begins as a small nodule. It grows rather slowly and in most cases ulcerates onto the surface. The most common appearance is a shallow ulceration with raised edges developed around the anal orifice, involving one or several quadrants. Some times the whole circumference of the anal orifice is involved (Fig. 35). Some squamous cell carcinomas of the anal margin are essentially exophytic, and may resemble benign condyloma. Only biopsy demonstrates their malignant nature.

Basal cell carcinoma of the anal margin may present as a flat, hard plaque with pearl-like nodules or pigmentation on the periphery, or as a rodent ulcer. This tumour is more common in males than in females. It is a local disease which spreads by direct extension, and does not tend to metastasize. Mixed basi-squamous cell carcinoma behaves as squamous cell carcinoma, and may give rise to lymphatic spread. Muco-epidermoid carcinoma may also be encountered. BOWEN's disease of the anal margin has recently been studied by STRAUSS and FAZIO (1979). It is a slow-growing intra-epithelial squamous cell cancer, usually involving large parts of the perineal area. It may resemble one of several different forms of chronic dermatosis. Usually, when the lesion has grown, it presents as a large, irregular, erythematous and pigmented zone of scaly, fissured plaques, which may extend laterally over a wide area. The epithelium is thickened, sometimes with definite tumour formation, which feels firm to the touch. Bowen's disease may be associated with other malignancies, which may already be present or may evolve at a later time. Perineal Paget's disease is excluded from this study, because it is an intra-epithelial adenocarcinoma.

The great variation in character of epidermoid carcicoma of the anal margin in its early stages is such that errors in diagnosis can be made. It can look like a simple erosion of the skin, or a fissure, or an unusual type of pile. However, cancer is harder and bleeds more easily than would be expected of a benign lesion (BENSAUDE and NORA 1968), and for any doubtful lesion a biopsy must be taken for diagnosis. When the tumour has grown larger, most cancers of the anal margin present as typical shallow ulceration with rolled, everted edges, firm to palpation, and there is no more difficulty in diagnosis.

2. Local Spread

The tumour grows mainly in the surface of the peri-anal region and may develop to a large extent in the direction of the buttocks or vulva. Most cancers of the anal margin remain outside the anal canal for a long period. If the lower anal canal is invaded, the involved area is usually very limited and concerns the superficial layers of the anal canal, sphincter muscles remaining free from cancer for a considerable time. The distinction between cancer of the anal margin invading the lower part of the anal canal and cancer of the anal canal involving the peri-anal skin is never a problem. At a later stage or when recurrence occurs after conservative treatment, the tumour may extend deeply into the underlying fatty structures of the perineum. Lymphatic spread to the inguinal and iliac nodes is observed in 15%–20% of cases. Distant metastases are rare.

3. Clinical Staging

The UICC pre-treatment clinical classification includes the following tumour categories, based on clinical examination, radiography, and endosdopy:

T_1 Tumour 2 cm or less in its greatest dimension, strictly superficial or exophytic

T_2 Tumour more than 2 cm but not more than 5 cm in its greatest dimension, or tumour with minimal infiltration of the dermis

T_3 Tumour more than 5 cm in its greatest dimension, or tumour with deep infiltration of the dermis

T_4 Tumour with extension to muscle, bone, etc.

Pre-treatment evaluation consists of a careful examination to determine the exact extent of the lesion in the perineal area and the anal canal, and the depth of invasion into the subcutaneous tissue. The limits of the tumour at the anal verge and in the lowest part of the anal canal must be clearly defined by endoscopy and rectal digital examination. When there is doubt, several biopsies should be taken at the border of the lesion, especially in the anal canal. The groins should be carefully palpated as part of a thorough general examination in all cases, and especially for Bowen's disease, having regard to the possibility of synchronous visceral tumour. Lymphangiography is required when inguinal lymph nodes are clinically involved.

4. Treatment

Epidermoid carcinoma of the anal margin shares the favourable prognosis of skin cancer, and should be treated conservatively with true preservation of the anal function for as long as possible. Although the lesion is known to be radiosensitive, local excision is the accepted treatment in many institutions "because of the undesirable effects of radiotherapy in the anal region". In these circumstances patients are referred to radiotherapy only under two conditions:
1. Inoperable, extensive, or recurrent lesion after conservative surgery
2. Operable lesion in patients who are not suitable candidates for surgery.

It is true that radionecrosis and fibrotic dystrophy may occur in the peri-anal area after high-dose irradiation. It is important to distinguish between benign, superficial necrosis easily curable without sequelae, and severe radionecrosis representing a major complication, most often suitable for radical surgery. Numerous advances have been made in the field of irradiation during the past decade to prevent not only the major but also the minor complications related to overdosage. At the present time, one can state that the development of radionecrosis after irradiation of a carcinoma of the peri-anal area is often due to a faulty technique, and should not follow correctly planned irradiation which has been delivered accurately. In other words, the respective roles of surgery and radiotherapy should be reconsidered.

a) Local Excision

Wide removal of the tumour has been described by STRAUSS and FAZIO (1979). It implies that an adequate margin can be secured between the growth and the normal tissue. In most squamous and basal cell carcinoma, the limits of the lesion are quite clearly defined, but with BOWEN's disease it is often impossible to determine the limits of the tumour on inspection; skin that appears to be perfectly normal may, in fact, be invaded by neoplasm. In such cases additional biopsies are taken at the periphery of the clinically involved area to define the limits of the area to be resected. All the involved skin is removed. GOLIGHER (1975) adds that it is customary to use surgical diathermy and to aim at a margin of clearance of at least 2.5 cm. In certain patients with Bowen's disease the skin of the entire circumference of the perineal and anal region, as well as the skin of the mucosa of the lower portion of the anal canal, has to be removed.

STRAUSS and FAZIO (1979) noticed that "if the surfaces are extensively denuded, they can be covered with a split-thickness skin graft. In such cases, the patients are put on a regimen of bed rest for one week and a clear liquid diet for five or seven days and are immediately given prescription to help prevent a bowel movement with subsequent fecal soilage of the graft." The length of stay in the hospital is short for patients with small tumour, but it may last more than a month for patients with large tumours requiring grafting.

There are very few reports of experience with epidermoid carcinomas of the anal margin, that is arising outside the anal verge (excluding the tumour arising in the lower portion of the anal canal). The most informative are the statistics of the Mayo Clinic published by Beahrs (1979). Of 31 cases, 27 were treated by local excision, four by irradiation. The survival rate was 74.2% at 5 years and 70.7% at 10 years.

At the Cleveland Clinic, AL-JURF et al. (1979) have reported ten previously untreated patients with squamous cell carcinoma of the peri-anal region who underwent local excision. Five patients were alive with no evidence of recurrence between 5 and 20 years post-operatively. One patient was alive but with recurrence after 6 years. One died of myocardial infarction 15 months post-operatively. Three relapsed after 3-4 months (two) and 6 years (one): two of these underwent further local excision, both being free from disease 12 years after the initial operation; and one underwent AP resection, with disclosed hypogastric lymph node metastases. This patient died 8 years after the initial operation. Seven additional patients presented with recurrent tumours. Two were treated palliatively for advanced relapses. Three underwent repeated local excision with complete long-term remission in two. Two patients underwent AP resection with or without radiotherapy; both were alive 9 years post-operatively. The authors concluded that selected patients with squamous cell carcinoma of the perineal area can be treated by local excision with excellent results.

The series of the St. Mark's Hospital was reported by HAWLEY (1980, personal communication). Of 70 patients seen between 1928 and 1974, 50 were treated by local excision, sometimes followed by irradiation; the 5-year survival rate was 60%. Twelve patients underwent an AP resection; five survived more than 5 years. Eight were treated by irradiation, four were cured. The overall 5-year survival rate was 55%.

b) Irradiation

Several modalities of irradiation can be used. Their effectiveness and their complication rates differ markedly (Table 33). Interstitial curietherapy with radium needles should be proscribed because the configuration of the peri-anal area does not allow good geometry of the radium implant, and especially because of the danger of radionecrosis if the size of the lesion exceeds 3 × 3 cm. MACCONNELL (1970) reported three severe complications in 12 cases so treated. Of 12 patients treated by radium implant at the Centre Léon Bérard between 1951 and 1970, three died of cancer – local extension (one), lymphatic spread (one), lung metastasis (one). Four died of intercurrent disease: five were alive and well at

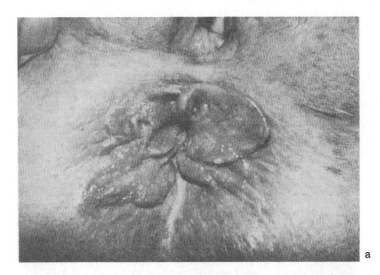

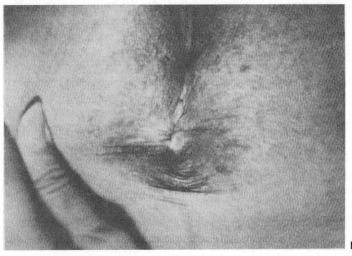

Fig. 35. a Epidermoid carcinoma of the external margin of the anus before treatment. The lesion is flat and has involved the whole circumference of the anal verge and the peri-anal area to some extent. **b** After irradiation with cobalt-60 at a given dose of 4200 rad in ten fractions within 16 days, the tumour has disappeared and is locally controlled. No necrosis or fibrosis

5 years; radionecrosis due to overdosage was observed in one patient. Interstitial curietherapy with iridium-192 can be applied with satisfactory parallelism of the wires in spite of the configuration of the anal margin. However it should only be used as a supplementary method after external irradiation with cobalt-60, which is by far the most efficient modality of irradiation for this type of tumour.

Protocol Used at the Centre Léon Bérard. Direct perineal irradiation with cobalt-60 has been discussed earlier, and has been shown to be efficient and well tolerated in the management of cancer of the anal canal. In the series of 27 patients treated since 1971, if one excepts a severe radionecrosis in one patient with a large infiltrating tumour treated in 1979, which required a permanent colostomy, no sequelae related to the cobalt itself have been seen. In all other cases, tolerance by the skin and subcutaneous tissue have been perfect, with no fibrosis of the perineal structure and preservation of a normal suppleness of the peri-anal area (Fig. 35).

Since 1971 the same technique of perineal irradiation has been the first approach in all patients with cancer of the anal margin: a given dose of 4000 rad is delivered in ten fractions of 400 rad over a period of 16 days. (The given dose is the maximum dose registered 5 mm beneath the surface).

The irradiation is applied in the manner described on p. 146, with the patient in the lithotomy position. The buttocks are taped apart so that the perineal area presents as flat an area as possible. The size on the field is adapted to the size of the lesion and encompasses an adequate margin around the pathological area. The usual dimensions are 7 × 7 cm to 10 × 10 cm. If the field exceeds 8 × 8 cm, the dose is reduced to 3600 rad, given dose.

The effectiveness of this radiation is reinforced by two means:
1. A combined short course fo chemotherapy is given according to the protocol of NIGRO et al. (1974) and of NEWMAN and QUAN (1976), sonsisting of 5-FU for the first 5 days of irradiation, and MTC for the 1st day (see p. 140).
2. When the tumour is flat and its thickness does not exceed 0.5 cm, a wax mould (bolus) 5 mm thick is applied over the surface of the tumoural area at the centre of the field of irradiation. Bolus is used every other application, that is in five of ten applications. It aims to prevent an underdosage to the superficial layers of the skin.

The irradiation with cobalt-60 is followed by a short period of skin and mucosal reaction, which does not last more than 10 days, and is followed by the shrinkage and disappearance of the tumour over 4–8 weeks. The treated area remains erythematous for 1 month and then returns to normal (Fig. 35a, b).

If a small residual focus of tumour remains at the end of the 2nd month, a booster dose of 2000 rad is given by interstitial curietherapy. The technique of after-loading iridium implant is the same as for any skin tumour. Plastic tubes or, preferably, steel needles are inserted (three or four lines, 10 mm apart) into the small target volume under general anaesthesia. Curietherapy increases the chance of local control without giving rise to necrotic complications, if it is applied with care. In the series of the Centre Léon Bérard, interstitial curietherapy as a supplementary method after cobalt therapy has been necessary in only four cases.

The protocol of cobalt therapy is easy to apply on an out-patient basis, whatever the age and the condition of the patient. Chemotherapy requires a short admission to hospital for 5 days. It is systematically applied except in very elderly, senile, debilitated patients.

All epidermoid carcinomas of the anal margin are suitable for such a protocol of irradiation, irrespective of size, degree of infiltration, extent to the anal canal, buttocks, or vulva, and histological type. This type of irradiation seems to be especially well adapted to treatment of Bowen's disease, because an adequate mar-

Table 33. Epidermoid carcinoma of the anal margin: Results of different modalities of treatment with irradiation[a]

Period of time	Treatment	No. of cases	Alive and well at 5 years	Deaths from cancer
1951–1970	Radium implant	12	5	3
1971–1977	Cobalt-60 ± iridium-192 ± chemotherapy (5-FU, MTC)	19	Alive and well at 4 years 12	3

[a] Centre Léon Bérard.

gin of normal skin is irradiated to prevent recurrences at the periphery of the lesion. However, there is one exception: for well-differentiated exophytic, condyloma-like lesions, a local excision with additive cobalt therapy seems to be a more successful approach.

Cobalt therapy (4000 rad given dose in 16 days) may also be used for elective post-operative treatment in the case of patients who have undergone local excision, when uncertainty remains about the complete removal of the neoplastic tissue.

Between 1971 and 1977 19 patients were seen and followed up for over 4 years. Their treatment consisted of cobalt therapy combined with iridium in four cases, and with chemotherapy (5-FU, MTC) in eight cases. Three died of cancer (two of nodal failures, one of lung metastases); four died of intercurrent disease. Twelve are alive and well, disease-free, more than 4 years later. Of the 19 patients only one had a local recurrence. No necrosis was observed.

5. Indications

a) Treatment of Tumours of the Anal Margin

All well-differentiated epidermoid carcinomas of the anal margin less than 3 cm in diameter, without infiltration, may be treated by local excision or by irradiation (cobalt + chemotherapy), as long as their margins are well defined and do not involve the lower part of the anal canal. However irradiation given by the protocol described has proved to be safer.

The rare, condyloma-like, well-differentiated carcinoma, limited in size, should be treated by local excision with elective post-operative cobalt therapy.

Irradiation is the most successful method for the following cases:
1. Large, superficial lesions more than 3 cm in diameter, whatever the histological type, or Bowen's disease
2. Lesions which have invaded the modified skin of the anal canal below the dentate line

3. Infiltrating tumours with involvement of underlying structures and inoperable, extensive tumours as well as recurrent lesions after local excision
4. Lesions in very elderly, handicapped patients, who represent a poor surgical risk.

   Chemotherapy (5-FU, MTC) is advisable as an adjuvant method if there are no contra-indications.

   However, these indications are valid only when irradiation is given by the techniques described in this chapter.

   The necessity for regular, frequent follow-up after conservative surgery or irradiation has been stressed before, and remains an essential condition after all types of conservative treatment.

   Radical surgery with permanent colostomy is only indicated when there is recurrent tumour unsuitable for local excision or irradiation.

b) Treatment of Inguinal Nodes

The general rules for the management of inguinal metastatic lymph nodes with cancer of the anal canal are also applicable to tumours of the anal margin. If mobile metastatic nodes are present when the patient is first seen, limited groin dissection with irradiation of both groins is indicated. If the metastatic lymph nodes are fixed and inoperable, high-dose irradiation is performed to control the lymphatic spread as well as the anal lesion. Prophylactic groin dissection is not advised when the patient agrees to regular follow-up. During this period, an inguinal node dissection should be done for local recurrence, and be followed by irradiation.

XVI. Conclusion

In oncology the optimal treatment is that which not only provides each patient with the best chance of control of cancer but also preserves the quality of life.

The management of cancer of the rectum has been the subject of much research during the past 2 decades. A better knowledge of the disease has helped to define new therapeutic approaches, which aim to increase survival rate and spare many patients permanent colostomy by using sphincter-saving procedures and conservative methods of treatment.

Substantial progress has been made in the detection of cancer of the rectum at an earlier stage. Pathological studies have identified a group of tumours with a low risk of lymph node involvement, which are suitable for conservative procedures as alternatives to radical surgery, particularly in poor-risk patients.

Local excision, electrocoagulation, and intracavitary irradiation are the three modalities of conservative therapy. The basic method of intracavitary irradiation is contact X-ray with the PHILIPS unit. It is an out-patient treatment requiring four to five applications within 6 weeks, easily applicable in all patients, and particularly suitable for elderly, frail, and debilitated patients. It may be combined with interstitial curietherapy by iridium-192. Applied to strictly selected patients, intracavitary irradiation has proved to have several advantages compared with local excision and electrocoagulation: higher rate of local control, lower occurrence of complications, and simplicity of application. Clinical and cytological follow-up is easy, with few false negatives and no problems when surgery is done for failure (207 patients have been followed up for more than 5 years with a rate of death from cancer of 10.6%).

In the selection of cases suitable for conservative treatment two points should be emphasized:
1. The importance of repeated clinical examination for metastatic lymph nodes in the mesorectum in patients with low rectal cancer (metastatic nodes found in 27 cases).
2. The place of elective inferior mesenteric and extra-mesenteric lymphadenectomy performed after control of the primary tumour in younger patients. This new surgical procedure may be considered as a safety measure and as an answer to the main objection to conservative procedures, which is the lack of knowledge about the presence of lymph node metastases.

Intracavitary irradiation also has a place:
1. In the treatment of cancer of the rectum located in the juxta-anal area in very poor risk patients. Such tumours are not suitable for conservative surgical procedures (44 cases).

Conclusion

2. As a supplementary treatment after local excision for malignant polyps to avoid further surgery (77 cases).
3. In the treatment of limited villous adenomas as definitive treatment, or for recurrence after local excision (70 cases).

Squamous cell carcinoma of the anal canal should not be treated by the same radical procedures as adenocarcinoma of the lower rectum because these diseases behave in very different ways.

For a long time irradiation therapy was only considered for the palliative treatment of inoperable patients, because of the high incidence of radionecrotic complications and treatment failures. However, important progress has been made in the field of irradiation, and the present approach to the treatment of carcinoma of the anal canal gives a prominent place to radiation therapy, which should be the first approach in all cases with or without subsequent surgery.

The background of this new approach considers the particular features of this disease: high radiosensitivity, perfect accessibility, danger of severe radionecrosis, slow pace of radiation response, and high incidence of pelvic lymph node involvement even at an early stage (metastatic nodes found in 50 cases).

Three protocols have been designed to deal with different clinical problems:
1. Curative irradiation given as combined external irradiation by cobalt-60 and interstitial curietherapy by iridium-192 in a split-course regimen. This protocol was applicable to about 75% of cases. Surgery was indicated after failure or necrosis (13.4%).
2. Pre-operative irradiation associated with chemotherapy (5-FU, MTC), followed by AP resection. This protocol is used for operable tumours not suitable for curative irradiation with preservation of anal function (fewer than 10% of patients).
3. High-dose pelvic irradiation for unresectable lesions, not suitable for curative surgery (15% of patients).

Treatment given along these lines controlled the disease in two out of three patients, and three-quarters of those cured were spared a permanent colostomy (121 cases followed up for over 3 years).

Epidermoid carcinoma of the anal margin is a skin cancer that originates in an area of particular importance because of the proximity to the anus and the susceptibility of the underlying structures to necrosis after irradiation. The first approach must be based on conservative treatment (31 patients have been followed up for more than 3 years).

Local excision or treatment by external irradiation with cobalt-60 will control localized tumours. Large or infiltrating tumours are suitable for external irradiation with cobalt-60 given carefully in a controlled manner. Radical surgery is only indicated when conservative treatment fails.

Irradiation given by intracavitary or external routes has a central role to play in the conservative treatment of cancers of the rectum and the anal canal and margin. But this treatment will only be successful when the protocols are planned carefully and supervised by a radiotherapist fully aware of his responsibility and working in close collaboration with a surgeon. In all cases the patient's agreement to careful and regular follow-up is an essential condition before conservative treatment is considered.

In the future, this collaboration will lead to improvement in the treatment of those patients suffering from these diseases, with the prospect of more cures with conservation of a normal sphincter.

XVII. References

A. Carcinoma of the Rectum

American Cancer Society (1979) Cancer journal for clinicians. Cancer 29:6–21
ASTLER VB, COLLER FA (1954) The prognosis significance of direct extension of carcinoma of the colon and rectum. Ann Surg 139:846–851
AXTELL LM, CUTLER SJ, MYERS MH (1972) End results in cancer. Report no. 4. HEW publication (NIH) 73–272:1

BABCOCK WW (1947) Radical single stage extirpation for cancer of the large bowel with retained functional anus. Sury Gynecol Obstet 85:1–7
BACON HE (1960) Major surgery of the colon and rectum: rehabilitation and survival rate in 2457 patients. Dis Colon Rectum 3:393
BACON HE (1964) Anus, rectum, sigmoid colon: diagnosis and treatment. Lippincott, Philadelphia
BEAHRS OH (1974) Status of fulguration and cryosurgery in the management of colonic and rectal cancer and polyps. Cancer 34:965–968
BERTILLON F, WERNER H (1933) A propos de la curiethérapie des cancers glandulaires inopérables du rectum. Bull Assoc Fr Cancer 22:591–605
BINKLEY CE (1928) Technical methods of radium application in rectal cancer. Am J Roentg 20:445–452, 1928.
BINKLEY CE (1938) Results of radiation therapy in primary operable rectal and anal cancer. Radiology 31:724–728
BLACK WA, WAUGH JM (1948) The intramural extension of carcinoma of the descending colon sigmoid and rectosigmoid. Surg Gynec Obstet 87:457–464
BOULIS-WASSIF S, HOP WCJ (1980) The role of preoperative adjuvant therapy in the management of borderline operability of rectal cancer. Coloproctology 2:320–326
BROMLEY JF (1938) Low-voltage, near-distance X-Ray therapy. Br J Radiol 11:289
BUGAT R, NGUYEN TD, EL SAFADI N, NAJA A, COMBES PF (1981) L'irradiation pré-opératoire des cancers du rectum. A propos d'une série de 96 cas. Bull Cancer (Paris) 68:363.
BUROKER T, NIGRO N, CORREA J, VAITKEVICIUS VK, SAMSON M, CONSIDINE B (1976) Combination preoperative radiation and chemotherapy in adenocarcinoma of the rectum. A preliminary report. Dis Colon Rectum 19:660–663

CADE S (1950) Malignant disease and its treatment by radium, 2nd edn. Simpkin Marshall, London
CARDEN ABG, MORSON BC (1964) Recurrence after local excision of malignant polyps of the rectum. Proc R Soc Med 57:559–561
CARTER S (1980) The contemporary management of anorectal cancer: selective alternatives. Symposium, Los Angeles, 21 Nov 1980
CARTER SK (1981) Adjuvant chemotherapy is of value in colon cancer. In Medical Oncology. Controversies in Cancer Treatment. Van Scoy-Mosher ed. Hall med. Publishers Boston Massachusetts.
CASS AW, MILLION RR, PFAFF WW (1976) Patterns of recurrence following surgery alone for adenocarcinoma of the colon and rectum. Cancer 37:2861–2865
CHAOUL H (1936) Die Behandlung operativ freigelegter Rektumkarzinome mit der Röntgennahbestrahlung. Munich Med Wochenschr 83:972
CHAOUL H, WACHSMANN F (1953) Die Nahbestrahlung. Thieme, Stuttgart

CHOLDINE SA (1955) Slokatchesvennie novaobrasovania priamoi kikhki. Med Leningrad Otdel, Leningrad
COHEN AM, GUNDERSON LL, WELCH CE (1981) Selective use of adjuvant radiation therapy in resectable colorectal adenocarcinoma. Dis Colon Rectum 24:247-251
CRILE G, TURNBULL RB (1972) The role of electrocoagulation in the treatment of carcinoma of the rectum. Surg Gynecol Obstet 135:391-396
CUGNENC P, GRASSIN P, PARC R, LOYGUE J (1981) Place et résultats de l'opération de Babcock dans le traitement du cancer du rectum à propos de 170 interventions. J Chir (Paris) 118:121-126
CULP CE (1976) Conservative management of certain selected cancers of the lower rectum. Controversy in surgery. Saunders, Philadelphia, 407-414
CULP CE, JACKMAN RJ (1974) Reappraisal of conservative management of certain selected cancers of the rectum. In: Najarian JS, Delaney JP (eds) Surgery of the gastrointestinal tract. Intercontinental Medical, New York 511-519

DUKES CE (1932) The classification of cancer of the rectum. J Pathol 35:323-332
DUKES CE (1940) Cancer of the rectum. An analysis of 1 000 cases. J Pathol Bacteriol 50:527
DUKES CE (1960) Cancer of the rectum. Livingstone, Edinburgh, London
DUKES CE, BUSSEY HJR (1950) The spread of rectal cancer and its effect on prognosis. Br J Cancer 12:309

EMANI B, WILLET C, PILE PRICH M, MILLER H (1979) Preoperative radiotherapy of unresectable colorectal carcimona. Int J Radiat Oncol Biol Phys [Suppl] 6:39
European Organisation for Research and Treatment of Cancer (EORTC) Brussels (1979) Protocol for controlled clinical trials for the treatment of patients with rectal cancer using surgery, radiotherapy and chemotherapy

FEIFEL G, LETZEL H (1980) Cryotherapy in rectal carcinoma. In: Welvaart K (ed) Colorectal cancer. Leiden University Press, The Hague 161-174
FINZI NS (1950) Report of meeting of the society of radiotherapists of Great Britain and Ireland, 15 May 1936. In: Cade S (ed) Malignant disease and its treatment by radium. Wright & Sons, London
FITZWILLIAMS DCL (1939) Inoperable carcinoma of the rectum. Lancet 2:675-678

GABRIEL WB (1969) The principles and practice of rectal surgery, 5th edn. HK Lewis, London
GABRIEL WB, DUKES CE, BUSSEY HJR (1935) Lymphatic spread in cancer of the rectum. Br J Surg 23:395
GARY-BOBO J, PUJOL J, SOLASSOL C, BROQUERIE J, NGUYEN M (1979) L'irradiation préopératoire du cancer rectal. Résultats à 5 ans de 116 cas. Bull Cancer (Paris) 66:491-496
GHOSSEIN NA, SAMALA EC, ALPERT S, DELUCA FR, RAGINS H, TURNER SS, STAGEY P, FLAX H (1981): Elective postoperative radiotherapy after incomplete resection of colorectal cancer. Dis Colon Rectum 24:252-256
GILBERTSEN VA (1960) Adenocarcinoma of the rectum: incidence and locations of recurrent tumor following present-day operations performed for cure. Am J Surg 151:340-348
GILCHRIST RK, DAVID VC (1947) A consideration of pathological factors influencing five-year survival in radical resection of the large bowel and rectum for carcinoma. Ann Surg 126:421
GOLIGHER JC (1976) The Dukes A, B and C categorization of the extent of spread of carcinomas of the rectum. Surg Gynecol Obstet 143:793-794
GOLIGHER JC (1977) Surgery of the anus, rectum and colon, 3rd ed., Charles C. Thomas, Springfield, IL.
GONDARD L (1951) A propos de 3 cas de carcinome rectal traités par contactherapie. J Electroradiol 32:743
GRINNELL RS, LANE N (1958) Benign and malignant adenomatous polyps and papillary adenomas of the colon and rectum. Int Abstr Surg:106-519
GUNDERSON L, SOSIN H (1974) Areas of failure found at reoperation (second or symptomatic look) following "curative surgery" for adenocarcinoma of the rectum. Cancer 34:1278-1292
GUNDERSON L, VOTAVA C, BROWN RC, PLENK HP (1976) Combined treatment with surgery and postoperative radiation LDS Hospital experience [Abstr]. Int J Radiat Biol Phys [Suppl] 1:64

HAWLEY PR, RITCHIE JK (1980) Indication technique and results of transanal tumour excision in cases of lower rectal carcinoma. In: REIFFERSCHEID H, LANGER S (eds) Der Mastdarmkrebs. Thieme, Stuttgart, pp 46–48

HELWIG EB (1947) Evolution of adenomas of large intestine and their relation to carcinoma. Surg Gynecol Obstet 84:36

HERMANEK P, ALTENDORF A, GUNSELMANN W (1980) Pathomorphologische Aspekte zu kontinenzerhaltenden Therapieverfahren bei Mastdarmkrebs. In: REIFFERSCHEID H, LANGER S (eds) Der Mastdarmkrebs. Thieme, Stuttgart, pp 1–12

HIGGINS GA (1977) Surgical considerations in colorectal cancer. Cancer 39:891–895

HIGGINS GA (1979) Adjuvant radiation therapy in colon cancer. Int Adv Surg Oncol 2:1–24

HIGGINS GA (1980) Preoperative radiation therapy for rectal carcinoma: Experience of the Veterans Administration surgical oncology group. Coloproctology 2:392–393

HIGGINS GA, ROSWIT B (1981) The role of radiotherapy in the surgical treatment of large bowel cancer. Prog Clin Cancer VII: 71–81

HIGGINS GA, CONN JA, JORDAN PH, HUMPHREY EW, ROSWIT B, KEEHN RJ (1975) Preoperative radiotherapy for colorectal cancer. Ann Surg 181:624–631

JACKMAN RJ (1961) Conservative management of selected patients with carcinoma of the rectum. Dis Colon Rectum 4:42

JACKSON BR (1977) Contemporary management of rectal cancer. Cancer 40:2365–2374

JACKSON BR (1980) Iridium implant in treatment of anorectal carcinoma. Dis Colon Rectum 23:145–150

JELDEN G, DHALIVAL R, LAVERY I, ANTONEZ AR, FAZIO V, LAVIK P, JAGELMAN D, WEAKLEY F, GAHBAVER R, HORTON J, THOMAS F, SANGHANI S (1981) Definitive treatment of rectal carcinoma with intracavitary radiation therapy. Int J Radiation Oncology Biol Physics 7, 1207

KLIGERMAN MM (1975) Preoperative radiation therapy in rectal cancer. Cancer 36:691–695

KLIGERMAN MM (1977) Radiotherapy and rectal cancer. Cancer 39:896–900

KNOCH HG, KOBERNICK H (1978) Kryochirurgische Behandlung des Anal-Rektum-Karzinoms. Zentralbl Chir 103:1420–1427

KOZLOVA AV, POPOVA TV (1977) Die Bedeutung der Strahlentherapie beim Rektumkarzinom. Radiobiol Radiother (Berl) 571–576

KRATZER GL, ONSANIT T (1972) Fulguration of selected cancers of the rectum, report of 27 cases. Dis Colon Rectum 15:431

LAMARQUE PL, GROS CG (1946) La radiothérapie de contact des cancers du rectum. J Radiol Electrol 27:333–348

LAMARQUE PL, GROS CG (1954) L'endoroentgenthérapie des cancers du canal anal et de l'ampoule rectale. J Electroradiol 35:245

LANGER S, BROCKAMP G (1980) Indikation, Technik und Ergebnisse der Kryotherapie beim Mastdarmkrebs. In: REIFFERSCHEID H, LANGER S (eds) Der Mastdarmkrebs. Thieme, Stuttgart

LARRÙ E (1957) Tratamiento del cancer del recto: Limites de accion eficaz en profundidad, de la roentgenterapia de chaoul por via peranal. Gac Med Esp 163–172

LOCALIO SA, ENG K, GOUGE TH, RANSON JHC (1978). Abdominosacral resection for carcinoma of the midrectum. Ten years experience. Annals of Surgery 188, 475–480

LOCK MR, CAIRNS DW, RITCHIE JK, LOCKHART-MUMMERY HE (1978) The treatment of early colorectal cancer by local excision. Br J Surg 65:346–349

LOCKHART-MUMMERY HE, DUKES CE (1952) Surgical treatment of malignant rectal polyps with notes on their pathology. Lancet 2:751

LOCKHART-MUMMERY HE, RITCHIE JK, HAWLEY PR (1976) The result of surgical treatment for carcinoma of the rectum at St Mark's Hospital from 1948 to 1972. Br J Surg 63:673–677

LOYGUE J, DUBOIS F (1966) Tumeurs malignes du rectum. Encycl Med Chir (Paris) [A] 10:9084-A10

MADDEN JL (1979) L'électrocoagulation dans le traitement du cancer du rectum. Chirurgie 105:15–24

MADDEN JL, KANDALAFT S (1967) Electrocoagulation. A primary and preferred method of treatment for cancer of the rectum. Ann Surg 106:413

MADDEN JL, KANDALAFT S (1971 a) Electrocoagulation in the treatment of the cancer of the rectum: a continuing study. Ann Surg 174:530

MADDEN JL, KANDALAFT S (1971 b) Clinical evolution of electrocoagulation in the treatment of the cancer of the rectum. Am J Surg 122:347

MAISIN J, LANGEROCK G (1953) Le traitement du cancer du rectum inopérable d'après 25 années de pratique hostpitalière à l'Institut du Cancer de Louvain. J Belge Radiol 36:335–356

MASON AY (1974) Transphincteric surgery of the rectum. In Prog Surg 13:66–97

MASON AY (1976a) Rectal cancer: the spectrum of selective surgery. Proc R Soc Med 69:237–244

MASON AY (1976b) Carcinoma of the lower two thirds of the rectum. Dis Colon Rectum 19:11–14

MASON AY (1977) Transphincteric approach to rectal lesions. Surg Annu 9:171–194

MASON AY (1980) Transphincteric surgery for lower rectal cancer. In: REIFFERSCHEID H, LANGER S (eds) Der Mastdarmkrebs. Thieme, Stuttgart, pp 39–45

MAYER M, BOBIN JY, PAPILLON J (1982). La lymphadénectomie mésentérique inférieure et extramésentérique dans le cancer du rectum. Chirurgie, Paris (to be published).

MILES WE (1926) Cancer of the rectum. Harrison, London

MOERTEL CG (1975) Clinical management of advanced gastrointestinal cancer. Cancer 36:675–682

MOHIUDDIN M, DOBELBOWER RR, KRAMER S, MARKS G (1981) Adjuvant radiotherapy with selective sandwich technique in treatment of rectal cancer. Results of continuing study. Dis Colon Rectum 24:76–79

MORGAN CN (1965) Carcinoma of the rectum. Ann R Coll Surg Engl 36

MORSON BC (1966) Factors influencing the prognosis of early cancer of the rectum. Proc R Soc Med 59:607–608

MORSON BC (1977) Polyps and cancer of the large bowel. In: YARDLEY JH, MORSON BC, ABELL MR (eds) The gastrointestinal tract [Int Acad Pathol Monogr]. Williams & Wilkins, BC, Baltimore, pp 101–108

MORSON BC (1979) Prevention of colorectal cancer. J R Soc Med 72:83–85

MORSON BC, BUSSEY HJR (1967) Surgical pathology of rectal cancer in relation to adjuvant radiotherapy. Br J Radiol 40:161

MORSON BC, VAUGMAN EG, BUSSEY HJR (1963) Pelvic recurrence after excision of rectum for carcinoma. Br Med J:13–18

MORSON BC, BUSSEY HJR, SAMOORIAN S (1977) Policy of local excision for early cancer of the colorectum. Gut 18:1045–1050

MOSS NH, AXTELL LM (1970) Cancers of gastrointestinal tract. Trends in methods of treatment. In: Lippincott (ed) Proceedings of the 6th national cancer conference. Philadelphia

MUIR EG (1960) The clinical diagnosis of rectal cancer. In: DUKES CE (ed) Cancer of the rectum. Livingstone, Edinburgh, London

NICHOLLS RJ, RITCHIE JK, WADSWORTH J, PARKS AG (1979) Total excision or restorative resection for carcinoma of the middle third of the rectum. Br J Surg 66:625–627

OSBORNE DR, HIGGINS AF, HOBBS KEF (1978) Cryosurgery in the management of rectal tumors. Br J Surg 65:859–861

PAPILLON J (1968) Place de l'irradiation dans le traitement conservateur des cancers limités du rectum et de l'anus. Acta Gastroenterol Belg 31:211–227

PAPILLON J (1973) Endocavitary irradiation of early rectal cancers: a series of 123 cases. Proc R Soc Med 66:1179–1181

PAPILLON J (1974) Endocavitary irradiation in the curative treatment of early rectal cancers. Dis Colon Rectum 172–180

PAPILLON J (1975a) Intracavitary irradiation of early rectal cancers for cure. A series of 186 cases. Cancer 36:696–701

PAPILLON J (1975b) Intracavitary irradiation of early rectal cancer for cure. Am J Proctol 37–41

PAPILLON J (1975c) Resectable rectal cancers. Treatment by curative endocavitary irradiation. JAMA 231:1385–1387

PAPILLON J (1977) Place de la radiothérapie intracavitaire à visée curative dans le traitement des cancers du rectum. Nouv Presse Med 6:250–254

PAPILLON J (1979) Intracavitary irradiation for cure of limited rectal cancers. General Surgery 2 13 A Harper and Row, London
PAPILLON J (1980a) Intracavitary irradiation for cure of limited rectal cancers. In: REIFFERSCHEID H, LANGER S (eds) Der Mastdarmkrebs. Thieme, Stuttgart
PAPILLON J (1980b) Le traitement des cancers limités du rectum par l'irradiation intracavitaire. Minerva Med 71:763-765
PAPILLON J (1981) Place de la radiothérapie à visée curative dans le traitement des adénocarcinomes du rectum et des carcinomes malpighiens du canal anal. Med Chir Dig 10:239-242
PAPILLON J, BAILLY C (1979) La recherche clinique des adénopathies et des nodules veineux métastatiques intra-pelviens dans l'évolution des cancers du bas rectum et du canal anal. Gastroenterol Clin Biol 3:600-601
PARKS AG (1972) Transanal technique in low rectal anastomosis. Proc R Soc Med 65:975
PARKS AG, THOMPSON JPS (1977) Per anal endorectal operative techniques in operative surgery. In: Todd IP (ed) Colon rectum and anus. Butterworth, London, pp 157-167
PARTURIER-ALBOT M (1965) La radiothérapie de contact des cancers du rectum. Indications et résultats. Ann Chir 19:1664
PARTURIER-ALBOT M (1979) Indications et résultats de la contacthérapie endocavitaire du cancer du rectum chez le sujet âgé. Ann Gastroenterol Hepatol 15:581-585
PATERSON R (1963) The treatment of malignant disease by radiotherapy. E Arnold, London
PIERQUIN B, CHASSAGNE DJ, CHAHBAZIAN CN, WILSON JF (1978) Brachytherapy. WH Green, St Louis
POIRIER A, POIRIER JP (1969) Electrodestruction dans les tumeurs malignes du rectum. Arch Fr Mal Appar Dig 58:37-48
POIRIER P, CUNEO B, DELAMERE G (1903) The lymphatics. Constable, London

RAYMOND A, HORIOT JC, GUILLAUD M, PAPILLON J, GUILLEMIN G (1977) Les tumeurs villeuses coliques et rectales. Analyse comparative du traitement chirurgical et du traitement radiothérapique. A propos de 104 observations. J Chir (Paris) 114:153-186
REE PC, MARKS JE, MOOSA AR, LEVIN B, PLATZ CE (1975) Rectal and rectosigmoid carcinoma: physician's prediction of local recurrence. J Surg Res 18:1-7
REGAUD C (1929) Radium therapy of the cancer at the radium institute of Paris; technique, biological principles and results. Am J Roentgenol 21:1
RENAUX R (1938) Cancer du rectum et radiothérapie. Monde Med 48:512-514
RIDER WD (1975) Is the Miles operation really necessary for the treatment of rectal cancer? J Can Assoc Radiol 26:167-175
ROMSDAHL M, WITHERS HR (1977) Adjuvant radiotherapy for carcinoma of the sigmoid colon and rectum. In: Salmon SE, Tones (eds) Adj therap cancer. Elsevier/North-Holland Biomedical Press, Amsterdam, pp 295-301
ROMSDAHL M, WITHERS HR (1978) Radiotherapy combined with curative surgery. Its use as therapy for carcinoma of the sigmoid colon and rectum. Arch Surg 113:446-453
ROSWIT B, HIGGINS GA (to be published) Primary and adjuvant radiotherapy in colorectal carcinoma. In: Mansfield C (ed) Therapeutic radiology. New directions in therapy. Medical Examination Publishing, Garden City, NY
ROSWIT B, HIGGINS G, HUMPHREY EW, ROBIHETTE CD (1973) Preoperative irradiation of operable adenocarcinoma of the rectum and recto-sigmoid colon. Radiology 108:389-395
ROUVIERE H (1932) Anatomie des lymphatiques de l'homme. Masson, Paris
RUBAY J, BOEUR JP (1978) Le traitement chirurgical du cancer du rectum. Acta Chir Belg 5:317-326
RUCKENSTEINER E (1954) Zur Nahbestrahlung des Anal und Rektalkarzinoms. Strahlentherapie 93:540
RUFF C, DOCKERTY M, FRICKE R, WAUGH J (1961) Preoperative radiation therapy for adenocarcinoma of rectum and rectosigmoid. Surg Gynecol Obstet 112:715-723

SALVATI EP, RUBIN RJ (1976) Electrocoagulation as primary therapy for rectal carcinoma. Am J Surg 132:583
SANFELIPPO PM, BEAHRS OH (1974) Carcinoma of the colon in patients under forty years of age. Surg Gynecol Obstet 138:169-170
SCHAEFER W, WITTE E (1932) Über eine neue Körperhöhlenröntgenröhre zur Bestrahlung von Uterustumoren. Strahlentherapie 44:283

SEEFELD PH, BARGEN JA (1943) The spread of carcinoma of the rectum: invasion of lymphatics veins and nerves. Ann Surg 118:76–90
SIMBERTSEVA LP, SNESHKO LI, SMIRNOV NM (1975) Results of intensive combined therapy for carcinoma of the rectum. Vopr Onkol 21:59
SIMSTEIN NL, KOVALCIK PL, CROSS GH (1978) Colorectal carcinoma in patients less than 40 years old. Dis Colon Rectum 21:169–171
SISCHY B, REMINGTON JH (1975) Treatment of cancer of the rectum by intracavitary irradiation. Surg Gynecol Obstet 562–564
SISCHY B, REMINGTON JH (1976) Endocavitary contact radiation for carcinoma of the rectum. Dis Colon Rectum 19:15–17
SISCHY B, REMINGTON JH, SOBEL SH (1978) Treatment of rectal carcinomas by means of endocavitary irradiation. Cancer 42:1073–1076
SISCHY B, REMINGTON JH, SOBEL SH, SAVLOV ED (1980a) Treatment of carcinoma of the rectum and squamous carcinoma of the anus by combination chemotherapy, radiotherapy and operation. Surg Gynecol Obstet 151:369–371
SISCHY B, REMINGTON JH, SOBEL S (1980b) Treatment of rectal carcinomas by means of endocavitary irradiation. Cancer 46:1957–1961
SMITH AN (1980) Radiotherapy in operable cancer of the rectum. Coloproctology 2:327–328
SPRATT TSJ, ACKERMAN LV (1962) Small primary adenocarcinomas of the colon and rectum. JAMA 179:337
STEARNS MWJ (1976) Limitations of local treatment of carcinoma of the rectum. Controversy in surgery. Saunders, Philadelphia
STEARNS MWJ, DEDDISH MR, QUAN SHQ (1959) Preoperative roentgentherapy for cancer of the rectum. Surg Gynecol Obstet 109:225–229
STEVENS K, ALLEN C, FLETCHER WS (1976) Preoperative radiotherapy for adenocarcinoma of the rectosigmoid. Cancer 37:2866–2874
STEVENS KRJ, FLETCHER WS, ALLEN CV (1977) A value of radiationtherapy for adenocarcinoma of the rectum and sigmoid. [Abstr] Digestion 16:278
STRAUSS AA (1969) Immunologic resistance to carcinoma produced by electrocoagulation, based on 57 years of experimental and clinical result. C Thomas, Springfield IL
STRAUSS AA, STRAUSS SF, CRAWFORD RA (1935) Surgical diathermy of carcinoma of the rectum, its clinical end results. JAMA 104:989–996
SWERDLOW DB, SALVATI FP (1972) Electrocoagulation of cancer of the rectum. Dis Colon Rectum 15:228
SWINTON NW, MOSZKOWSKI E, SNOW JC (1959) Cancer of the colon and rectum: A statistical study of 608 patients. Surg Clin North Am 39:475
SYED AMN (1975) Management of extensive residual cancer with interstitial iridium implant. A preliminary report. In: Hilaris (ed) After loading 20 years of experience, 1955–1975. Memorial Sloan-Kettering Cancer Center, New York, pp 119–124
SYED AMN, FEDER BH (1977) Technique of after loading interstitial implants. Radiol Clin (Basel) 46:458–475
SYED AMN, PUTHAWALA A, NEBLETT D, GEORGE FW III., MYINT US, LIPSETT JA, JACKSON BR, FLEMMING PA (1978) Primary treatment of carcinoma of the lower rectum and anal canal by a combination of external irradiation and interstitial implant. Radiology 128:199–203
SYMONDS CJ (1913–1914) Cancer of the rectum: excision after application of radium. Proc R Soc Med 7:153

TODD J (1968) Treatment of cancer of the rectum and anal region by local surgery. Act Gastroenterologia Belg 31:228–231
TURNBULL RBJ (1974) Carcinoma of the rectum. Nonresective treatment. Dis Colon Rectun 17:588–590
TURNBULL RBJ (1975) The no touch isolation technique of resection. JAMA 231:1181
TURNBULL RBJ, CUTHBERTSON AM (1961) Abdominorectal pull through resection for cancer and for Hirschsprung's disease. Cleve Clin Q 28:109
TURNER SS, VIEIRA EP, GAER PJ et al. (1977) Elective postoperative radiotherapy for locally advanced colorectal cancers. Cancer 40:105

VAN DER PLAATS GJ (1938) Die Röntgenkaustik, ihre Grundsätze und ihre Anwendung. Strahlentherapie 61:84
VAN SLOOTEN EA, VAN DOBBENBURGH OA (1980) Electrofulguration for rectal cancer. In: WELVAART K (ed) Colorectal cancer. Leiden University Press, The Hague, pp 175–180
VILLACEQUE R, BRANELLEC R, FATBISOWICZ S (1962) Orientation thérapeutique dans les cancers anorectaux à l'institut Gustave Roussy. Gaz Med Fr 23:163
VILLEMIN F, HUARD P, MONTAGNE (1925) Recherches anatomiques sur les lymphatiques du rectum et de l'anus. Rev Chir 39:63

WANEBO HJ, QUAN SHQ (1979) Failures of electrocoagulation of primary carcinoma of the rectum. Surg Gynecol Obstet 138:174–176
WANG CC, SCHULZ MD (1962) The role of radiation therapy in the management of carcinoma of the sigmoid, rectosigmoid and rectum. Radiology 79:1–5
WATERHOUSE JAH, MUIR CS, CORREA P, POWELL J (eds) (1976) Cancer incidence in five continents, vol III, publ 15. International Agency for Research on Cancer, Lyon
WEBB AJ (1979) Cytology diagnosis of anorectal and rectosigmoid lesions by a simple smear technique. Acta Cytol (Baltimore) 23:524
WILLIAMS IG, HORWITZ H (1956) The primary treatment of adenocarcinoma of the rectum by high voltage roentgen-rays (1000 kV). Am J Roentgenol 76:919–928
WILSON E (1973) Local treatment of cancer of the rectum. Dis Colon Rectum 16:194–199
WITHERS HR, ROMSDAHL MM, BARKLEY HT, SAXTON J, MC BRIDE C, MC MURTREY M, (1979) Postoperative radiotherapy as an adjuvant to surgical resection of adenocarcinoma of the rectum and recto-sigmoid. Meeting Abstract of the 2d International Conference on the Adjuvant Therapy of Cancer, March 28–31, Tucson, Arizona
WHITTAKER M, GOLIGHER JC (1976) The prognosis after surgical treatment for carcinoma of the rectum. Br J Surg 63:384–388
WITTOESCH JH, JACKMAN RJ (1958) Results of conservative management of cancer of the rectum in poor risk patients. Surg Gynecol Obstet 107:648

ZUCALI R, GARDANI G, VOLTERRANI F (1980) Adjuvant postoperative radiotherapy in locally advanced rectal and rectosigmoid cancer. Tumori 66:595–600

B. Carcinome of the Anus

AL-JURF AS, TURNBULL RB, FAZIO VW (1979) Local treatment of squamous cell carcinoma of the anus. Surg Gynecol Obstet 148:576

BACON HE (1964) Cancer of the colon, rectum and anal canal. Lippincott, Philadelphia
BEAHRS OH (1979) Management of cancer of the anus. Am J Roentgenol 133:791–795
BEAHRS OH, WILSON SM (1976) Carcinoma of the anus. Ann Surg 184:422–428
BENSAUDE A, NORA J (1968) Differential diagnosis of carcinoma of the anal margin. Proc R Soc Med 61:624–626
BOND WH (1960) Discussion on squamous cell carcinoma of the anus and anal canal. Proc R Soc Med 53:411
BRENNAN JT, STEWART CF (1972) Epidermoid carcinoma of the anus. Ann Surg 176:78
BROWN DA, MCKENZIE AD (1963) Squamous cell carcinoma of the anus. Can J Surg 61:629
BRUCKNER HW, SPIGELMAN MK, MANDEL E et al. (1979) Carcinoma of the anus treated with a combination of radiotherapy and chemotherapy. Cancer Treat Rep 63:395–398

CHRUSCOV MM, SEMAKINA ER, RAIFEL BA (1978) Radiotherapy for rectal epidermoid carcinoma. Radiobiol Radiother (Berl) 19:685–689
CORMAN ML, HAGGITT RC (1977) Carcinoma of the anal canal. Surg Gynecol Obstet 145:674–676
COURTIAL J, FERNANDEZ COLMEIRO JM (1960) Les indications et les résultats de la roentgenthérapie et de la curiethérapie dans le cancer du canal anal. Arch Mal Appar Dig 49:43
CUMMINGS BJ, HARWOOD AR, KEANE TJ, THOMAS GM, RIDER WD (1980) Combined treatment of squamous-cell carcinoma of the anal canal. Dis Colon Rectum 23:389–391

DALBY JE, POINTON RS (1961) The treatment of anal carcinoma by intersitial irradiation. Am J Roentgenol 85:515
DARGENT M (1958) Le cancer de l'anus. Rev Prat 8:731–741
DEVOIS A, DECKER R (1960) La curiepuncture du cancer de l'anus. Arch Fr Mal Appar Dig 49:54
DILLARD BM, SPRATT JS, ACKERMAN LV, BUTCHER HR (1963) Epidermoid cancer of anal margin and canal. Review of 79 cases. Arch Surg 86:772
DUKES CE (1960) Cancer of the rectum. Livingstone, Edinburgh, London

ESCHWEGE F, FAJBISOWICZ S, OTMZGUINE Y, SARRAZIN D (1973) Cancers épidermoides de l'anus. J Radiol Electrol 54:636
ESCHWEGE F, BRETEAU N, CHAVY A, LASSER P, WIBAULT P, KAC J (1979) Complication de la radiothérapie transcutanée des épithéliomas du canal anal. Gastroenterol Clin Biol (Paris) 3, 183–186

GABRIEL WD (1941) Squamous cell carcinoma of anus and anal canal. Proc R Soc Med 34:139
GILLESPIE JJ, MACKAY B (1978) Histogenesis of cloacogenic carcinoma. Hum Pathol 9:579–587
GOLDEN CT, HORSLEY JS (1976) Surgical management of epidermoid carcinoma of the anus. Am J Surg 131:275–280
GOLIGHER JC (1975) Surgery of the anus, rectum and colon, 3rd edn. C Thomas, Springfield IL
GRINNELL RS (1954) An analysis of forty-nine cases of squamous cell carcinoma of the anus. Surg Gynecol Obstet 98:29–39
GRINVALSKY HT, HELWIG EB (1956) Carcinoma of the ano-rectal junction. Cancer 9:480–488

HARDCASTLE JD, BUSSEY JR (1968) Results of surgical treatment of squamous cell carcinoma of anal canal and anal margin. St Mark's Hospital. Proc R Soc Med 61:629
HARDY KJ, HUGHES ESR, CUTHBERTSON AM (1969) Squamous cell carcinoma of the anal canal and anal margin. Aust NZ J Surg 38:301–305
HERMANN G, DESFOSSES L (1880) Sur la muqueuse de la région cloacale du rectum. CR Acad Sci (Paris) 90:1–30
HIGHTOWER BM, JUDD ES (1967) Carcinoma of canal anal and anus therapy. Mayo Clin Proc 42:271
HOLMES EC, MOSELEY HS, MORTON DL, CLARK W, ROBINSON D, URIS MM (1977) A rational approach to the surgical management of melanoma. Ann Surg 186:481–490
HOHM WH, JACKMAN RJ (1964) Anorectal squamous cell carcinoma. Conservative or radical treatment. JAMA 188:162–172

JACKSON BR (1980) Iridium implant in treatment of anorectal carcinoma. Dis Colon Rectum 23:145–150
JUDD ES Jr, DE TAR BE Jr (1955) Squamous cell carcinoma of the anus: Results of treatment. Surgery 37:220

KEILING R, GRUNEWALD JM, ACHILLE E (1973) La curiethérapie interstitielle à l'iridium 192 des épithéliomas du canal anal. J Radiol Electrol 54:634–635
KLOTZ RG, PAMUKOGLU T, SOUILLARD DH (1967) Transitional cloacogenic carcinoma of the anal canal. Clinicopathological study of 373 cases. Cancer 20:1727–1745
KUEHN PG, EISENBERG H, REED JF (1968) Epidermoid carcinoma of the perianal skin and anal canal. Cancer 22:932–938

LOYGUE J, LAUGIER A, PARC R, WEISGERBER G (1981) Carcinome épidermoïde de l'anus, à propos de 149 observations. Chirurgie 109:710

MACCONNELL EM (1970) Squamous carcinoma of the anus: a review of 96 cases. Br J Surg 57:89–92
MOLLER C (1970) Cancer of the anus and anal canal. Acta Chir Scand 136:340–348
MORSON BC (1960) The pathology and results of treatment of squamous cell carcinoma of the anal canal and anal margin. Proc R Soc Med 53:416–420
MORSON BC, PANG LSC (1968) Pathology of anal cancer. Proc R Soc Med 61:623–624
MORSON BC, SOBIN LH (1964) Histological classification of intestinal tumours. WHO, Geneva

NEWMAN HK, QUAN SH (1976) Multimodality therapy for epidermoid carcinoma of the anus. Cancer 37:12–19

References

NIGRO MD, VAITKEVICIUS VK, CONSIDINE BJ (1974) Combined therapy for cancer of the anal canal. A preliminary report. Dis Colon Rectum 17:354

NIGRO MD, VAITKEVICIUS VK, BUROKER T, BRADLEY GT, CONSIDINE BJ (1981) Combined therapy for cancer of the anal canal. Dis Colon Rectum 24:73–75

O'BRIEN JP, LOMBARDO SS, OPPENHEIM A (1950) Carcinoma of the anus. Am J Surg 79:832–833

PACK GT, REKERS P (1942) The management of malignant tumors in the groin. Am J Surg 56:545–565

PAPILLON J (1968) Place de l'irradiation dans le traitement conservateur des cancers limités du rectum et de l'anus. Acta Gastroenterol Belg 31:211–227

PAPILLON J (1974) Radiation therapy in the management of epidermoid carcinoma of the anal region. Dis Colon Rectum 17:184–187

PAPILLON J (1976) Place de la radiothérapie à visée curative dans le traitement des cancers du bas rectum et des cancers du canal anal. J Med Lyon 57:573–582

PAPILLON J, BAILLY C (1979) La recherche clinique des adénopathies et des nodules veineux métastatiques intrapelviens dans l'évolution des cancers du bas rectum et du canal anal. Gastroenterol Clin Biol 3:600–601

PAPILLON J, GERARD JP (1975) Cancer de l'anus. Encycl Med Chir Ther 25 575 C10

PAPILLON J, MONTBARBON JF, CHASSARD JL, GERARD JP, JAUSSAUD D (1973) Place de la curiethérapie seule ou combinée à la cobalthérapie dans le traitement des cancers épidermoïdes de l'anus. J Radiol Electrol 54:627–633

PAPILLON J, MONTBARBON JF, GERARD JP, CHASSARD JL (1979) Les radionécroses après curiethérapie des carcinomes épidermoides de l'anus. Gastroenterol Clin Biol 3:193–198

PAPILLON J, MAYER M, MONTBARBON JF, CHASSARD JL, GERARD JP, BAILLY C, TOURAINE-ROMESTAING P (1980) Le cancer du canal anal en 1980. Nouvelle approche thérapeutique. Concours Med 102:3373–3383

PARADIS P, DOUGLAS HJ, HOLYORE ED (1975) The clinical implications of a staging system for carcinoma of the anus. Surg Gynecol Obstet 141:411–416

PARKS A (1981) Squamous carcinoma of the anal canal. Ann Gastroenterol Hepatol 17:103–107

PILLERON JP, ROUSSEAU J, DEBERTRAND P, DURAND JC, MATHIEU G, DESCHAMPS P (1970) 286 cas de cancer du canal anal. Place de la chirurgie et de la cobalthérapie. Mem Acad Chir 96:143–151

PILLERON JP (1973) La chirurgie dans le traitement du cancer du canal anal. J Radiol Electrol 54:620–621

QUAN SHQ (1978a) Anal and para-anal tumors. Surg Clin North Am 58:591–603

QUAN SHQ (1978b) Treatment of anal cancer. 1er congrès mondial de proctologie, Madrid, Mai 1978

QUAN SHQ (1979) Squamous cancer of the anorectum. Int J Radiat Oncol Biol Phys 5:63

QUAN SHQ, GORDON B, MAGILL MD, LEAMING RM, MAJDU SI (1978) Multidisciplinary preoperative approach to the management of epidermoid carcinoma of the anus and anorectum. Dis Colon Rectum 21:89–91

RAVEN RW (1941) Squamous-cell carcinoma of the anus and anal canal. Proc R Soc Med 34:157

RICHARDS JC, BEAHRS OH, WOOLNER LB (1962) Squamous-cell carcinoma of anus, anal canal and rectum in 109 patients. Surg Gynecol Obstet 114:475

ROUSSEAU J, MATHIEU G, FENTON J, CUZIN J (1973) La télécobalthérapie des cancers du canal anal. J Radiol Electrol 54:622–626

ROUSSEAU J, MATHIEU G, FENTON J (1979) Resultats et complications de la radiothérapie des epitheliomas du canal anal. Etude de 128 cas traités de 1956 a 1970. Gastroenterol Clin Biol (Paris) 3:207–208

ROUX-BERGER JL, ENNUYER A (1948) Carcinoma of the anal canal. Am J Roentgenol 60:807

SAWYERS JL (1972) Squamous cell carcinoma of the perianus and anus. Surg Clin North Am 52:935–941

SAWYERS JL, HERRINGTON JL, MAIN BF (1963) Surgical consideration in the treatment of epidermoid carcinoma of the anus. Ann Surg 157:817

SEDGWICK CE, WAINSTEIN E (1959) Epidermoid carcinoma of the anus and rectum. Surg Clin North Am 39:759

STEARNS MW, QUAN SH (1970) Epidermoid carcinoma of the anorectum. Surg Gynecol Obstet 131:953–957

STRAUSS RJ, FAZIO VW (1979) Bowen's disease of the anal and perianal area: a report and analysis of twelve cases. Am J Surg 137:231–234

SVENSON EW, MONTAGUE ED (1980) Results of treatment in transitional cloacogenic carcinoma. Cancer 46:828–830

SWEET RH (1947) Results of treatment of epidermoid carcinoma of the anus and rectum. Surg Gynecol Obstet 84:967–972

WANEBO HJ, CONSTABLE WC, FUTRELL JW, ROSENOFF S (1980) A multimodality approach to the surgical management of locally advanced epidermoid carcinoma of the anorectum. Proc Am Assoc Cancer Res 21:417

WANEBO HJ, FUTRELL JW, CONSTABLE WC, ROSENOFF S (1981) Multimodality approach to the surgical management of locally advanced epidermoid carcinoma of the anorectum. Cancer 47:2817–2829

WELCH JP, MALT RA (1977) Appraisal of the treatment of carcinoma of the anus and anal canal. Surg Gynecol Obstet 145:837–841

WILLIAMS IG (1962) Carcinoma of the anus and anal canal. Clin Radiol 13:30–34

WOLFE HRI (1968) The management of metastasis inguinal adenitis in epidermoid cancer of the anus. Proc R Soc Med 61:626–628

XVIII. Subject Index

Cancer of the Rectum

Accessibility 98
Age 6
Astler-Coller classification 17

Bleeding 80

CEA level 29
Clinical staging 41
Colloid carcinoma 8
Conservative irradiation 63
Conservative procedures 38
– –, selection 40
– –, mode of action 100
– –, control of tumour 101
Contact X-ray therapy 66, 75
Cryosurgery 61
Cytology (role of) 89

Distant metastases 17, 86, 89
Dosimetry of Curietherapy 74
Dukes' Classification 17
Dysplasia-carcinoma sequence 10

Early cancer 9
Electrocoagulation 56
– and irradiation 56
– (Mayo Clinic) 57
– (Cleveland Clinic) 58
– (St Clare's Hospital) 59
Extra mural spread 12

Fistula (recto-vaginal) 102
Follow-up 51, 88, 103
Frequency 5
Fulguration 56

GITSG trial 34

Haemoccult test 7
Histological grading 9, 15, 77
Histology 8
Hypogastric lymph nodes 14

Interstitial curietherapy 70, 99
Intracavitary irradiation 75
Intracavitary irradiation (indications) 98
Intramural spread 11
Iridium 192 13, 99

Juxta-anal rectal cancer 95

Knee-chest position 44, 73, 77

Liver metastases 17
Local excision 52
– –, selection 54
– – and irradiation 105
Local failures 89
Local spread and cure rate 13
Lymphadenectomy 47
Lymphatic spread 13
– – and histological grading 14
– – and local spread 14
– – and prognosis 15

Mortality after surgery 22
Muscular layers (invasion) 12, 17

No touch isolation technique 24
Nodal failures 91

Overlapping fields 79, 92

Palpable metastatic pelvic nodes 45, 91, 98
Pararectal lymph nodes 14
Perforation 102
Polyp-cancer sequence 10
Polypoid cancer 12, 80, 99
Postoperative irradiation 33
– –, technique 35
Pre-operative irradiation 24
– –, selection 27
– –, protocol 29
– – and chemotherapy 32
Pull-through procedures 20

Radical surgery 21
Radiocurability 83
Radionecrosis 83
Radiosensibility 83
Recurrence 88
Resectability 22
Response to radiation 80
Restorative procedures 21

Sandwich technique 35
Scrape smears cytology 89
Search for pelvic nodes 45, 91, 98
Sexual dysfunction 23
Shrinkage after irradiation 80
Spread 13
Staging 17

Stapling devices 20
Surgery-results 20

Third week test 43
Topographical distribution 6
Total biopsy 100
Trans-sphincteric operation 52
Treatment applicators 77

Ulcerative carcinoma 10, 11, 80, 99
Urinary complications of surgery 23

Venous spread 16
Venous spread and local spread 16
Villous adenomas 12, 105

Wedge filter 31, 37

Cancer of the Anus

Accessibility 138
Adenocarcinoma 113
After loading 150
Age 114
Anal crypts 113
Anal margin carcinoma 178
Anatomy of anal area 111
Arctherapy 146
Aspiration biopsy for inguinal modes 123, 174

Basal cell carcinoma 178
Basaloid carcinoma 112
Bolus (wax) 183
Bowen's disease 180

Cloacogenic carcinoma 112
Cobalt 60 135, 146, 151, 163, 183
Colloid carcinoma 113
Colostomy 130
Configuration 115
CT Scan 124
Cytology 123, 159

Dentate line 111
Diagnosis 121
Dosimetry 150
Distant spread 121

Electrons 174
External beam irradiation 133, 146

Fibrotic dystrophy 137
Fractionation 144

Frequency 114
Fluorouracile 141, 156, 183

Groin dissection (see inguinal dissection)

Haemorrhoids 115, 121
Histology 112, 178
Hypogastric lymph nodes 119

Inguinal area irradiation 163, 175
Inguinal nodes (first symptom) 121, 122
Inguinal nodes 118, 123, 162, 175
Inguinal dissection 163, 173
Internal iliac chain 119
Interstitial curietherapy 132, 148, 183
Iridium 192 implant 148, 151, 170, 176, 184
Isodose distribution 147, 150, 155

Knee-chest position 122

Late diagnosis 121
Liver scan 124
Local excision 126
Local failures 158, 180
Local spread 116
Lymphadenectomy (pelvic) 168, 176
Lymphangiography 123
Lymphatic spread 117

Major surgery (MILES) 127
Metachronous node metastasis 164
Metastasis 121, 179
Middle hemorrhoidal chain 119
Mitomycin C 141, 156, 183

Subject Index

Mortality (operative) 128
Mucoepidermoid carcinoma 111, 178
Multimodality treatment 141

Pace of shrinkage 139
Pectinate line 111
Pelvic irradiation 161
Pelvic nodal failures 160, 176
Pelvic node (first symptom) 123, 167
Pelvic lymph nodes 120, 160, 175
Perianal skin 173
Perineal field 146
Preoperative irradiation 142, 154
Preoperative radio-chemotherapy 141, 172
Presacral irradiation 146

Radionecrosis 136, 139, 189
Radiosensitivity 138
Radium implant 131, 181
Rectovaginal wall 117
Rectovaginal fistula 121, 137

Search for pelvic nodes 123, 164, 176
Sex ratio 115
Silver grain 149

Site 111
Split-course irradiation 143
Spread 116, 160, 179
Squamous-cell carcinoma 112, 178
Staging 124, 179
Superior haemorrhoidal chain 119
Surgery (radical) 127
Surgery (extended) 130
Symptoms 121
Synchronous node metastases 164, 167

Template for Iridium implant 148
Time factor 139
TNM classification 124, 179
Tolerance 151
Transitional carcinoma 112
Transitional zone 112

Unresectable tumours 145, 161, 172

Vaginal examination 123
Venous spread 104

Wedge filter 147, 154

Colorectal Cancer

Editor: W. Duncan

1982. 50 figures, 51 tables. X, 156 pages
(Recent Results in Cancer Research, Volume 83)
ISBN 3-540-11395-9

Contents: Recent Trends. – Aetiology. – Cell Kinetics. – Relevance of Colonic Mucosal Inflammation to the Aetiology. – Genetic Factors. – Pathology and Natural History. – Biochemical Markers. – Radiological Assessment. – Early Diagnosis and Detection. – Surgery. – Radiotherapy. – Chemotherapy. – Prospects in Management. – Subject Index.

A multidisciplinary account of our understanding and management of colorectal cancer is provided in this volume. The aetiology of the disease is reviewed and the factors associated with its high incidence in affluent Western societies are described. Accounts are given of new aspects of the pathology of the disease and of radiological and biochemical factors. The importance of early diagnosis is stressed, and the development of techniques in this area are given in detail. Current trends in management by surgery, radiotherapy and chemotherapy are described, with particular reference to the large number of clinical trials that have been conducted throughout the world.

Colo-rectal Surgery

Editors: G. Heberer, H. Denecke

1982. 91 figures, 89 tables. 220 pages
ISBN 3-540-11505-6

The current status of colorectal surgery is discussed in this book by leading specialists from Europe and Australia. Orginally presented at the Anglo-German Proctology Meeting, their contributions reflect not only results in clinical treatment, but also research issues in pathology, anatomy and experimental surgery.
Among the topics covered in this work are
- the megacolon as a symptom of various etiology including Hirschsprung's disease, constipation, idiopathic megacolon, and pseudoobstruction
- rectal anal anastomoses, with special emphasis on suture techniques
- the surgical, radiologic and multimodality treatment of anal carcinoma
- sphincter disfunction and hemorrhoids, and special aspects of inflammatory disease.

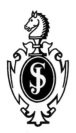

Springer-Verlag
Berlin
Heidelberg
New York

Recent Results in Cancer Research

Fortschritte der Krebsforschung
Progrès dans les recherches sur le cancer

Editor in Chief: P. Rentchnick
Co-editor: H. J. A. Senn
discount of 20 per cent on list price is granted to those purchasing the complete series

A Selection

Volume 67
Adjuvant Therapies and Markers of Post-Surgical Minimal Residual Disease I
Markers and General Problems of Cancer Adjuvant Therapies
Editors: G. Bonadonna, G. Mathé, S. E. Salmon
1979. 64 figures, 40 tables. XVIII, 150 pages
ISBN 3-540-09291-9

Volume 68
Adjuvant Therapies and Markers of Post-Surgical Minimal Residual Disease II
Adjuvant Therapies of the Various Primary Tumors
Editors: G. Bonadonna, G. Mathé, S. E. Salmon
1979. 181 figures, 218 tables. XI, 465 pages
ISBN 3-540-09360-5

Volume 69
Strategies in Clinical Hematology
Editors: R. Gross, K.-P. Hellriegel
1979. 22 figures, 33 tables. X, 140 pages. (Book of Main Lectures – 5th Meeting of the European and African Division of the International Society of Haematology/Hamburg, August 26th – 31th, 1979)
ISBN 3-540-09578-0

Volume 70
New Anticancer Drugs
Editors: S. K. Carter, Y. Sakurai
1980. 83 figures, 164 tables. XI, 229 pages
ISBN 3-540-09682-5

Volume 74
Cancer Chemo- and Immunopharmacology I
Chemopharmacology
Editors: G. Mathé, F. M. Muggia
1980. 82 figures, 150 tables. XIII, 315 pages
ISBN 3-540-10162-4

Volume 75
Cancer Chemo- and Immunopharmacology II
Immunopharmacology, Relations and General Problems
Editors: G. Mathé, F. M. Muggia
1980. 76 figures, 83 tables. XI, 260 pages
ISBN 3-540-10163-2

Volume 76
New Drugs in Cancer Chemotherapy
Editors: S. K. Carter, Y. Sakurai, H. Umezawa
1981. 133 figures, 170 tables. XIV, 336 pages
(U. S. Japan Joint Agreement on Cancer Research 5th Annual Program Review Symposium, San Francisco (USA), May 21–22, 1979)
ISBN 3-540-10487-9

Volume 77: K. E. Stanley, J. Stjernswärd, M. Isley
The Conduct of a Cooperative Clinical Trial
1981. 9 figures, 13 tables. XI, 75 pages
ISBN 3-540-10680-4

Volume 79
Chemotherapy and Radiotherapy of Gastrointestinal Tumors
Editor: H. O. Klein
1981. 38 figures, 59 tables. VII, 112 pages
ISBN 3-540-10938-2

Volume 80
Adjuvant Therapies of Cancer
Editors: G. Mathé, G. Bonadonna, S. Salmon
1982. 68 figures, 116 tables. XII, 356 pages
ISBN 3-540-10949-8

Volume 81: H.-P. Lohrmann, W. Schreml
Cytotoxic Drugs and the Granulopoietic System
1981. 6 figures, 87 tables. VIII, 222 pages
ISBN 3-540-10962-5

Springer-Verlag
Berlin
Heidelberg
New York

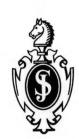

Printed by Publishers' Graphics LLC
DBT131103.20.05.52 20131103